DUAL DIAGNOSIS

Second Edition

DUAL DIAGNOSIS

Counseling the Mentally Ill Substance Abuser

Second Edition

KATIE EVANS
J. MICHAEL SULLIVAN

THE GUILFORD PRESS
New York   London

© 2001 The Guilford Press
A Division of Guilford Publications, Inc.
72 Spring Street, New York, NY 10012
www.guilford.com

Printed in the United States of America

This book is printed on acid-free paper.

Last digit is print number: 9 8 7 6 5 4 3 2 1

Library of Congress Cataloging-in-Publication Data

Evans, Katie.
    Dual diagnosis : counseling the mentally ill substance abuser / Katie Evans,
J. Michael Sullivan.—2nd ed.
      p. cm.
    Includes bibliographical references and index.
    ISBN 1-57230-446-4 (pbk.)
      1. Dual diagnosis—Patients—Counseling of. I. Sullivan, J. Michael.
II. Title.
    RC564.68 .E95 2001
    616.86—dc21   00-063637

The Twelve Steps and excerpts from pp. 58–60 and 499 from the book *Alcoholics
Anonymous* are reprinted with permission of Alcoholics Anonymous World Services,
Inc. (AAWS). Permission to reprint the Twelve Steps and these excerpts does not
mean that AAWS has reviewed or approved the contents of this publication, or that
AAWS necessarily agrees with the views expressed herein. AA is a program of recovery
from alcoholism *only*—use of the Twelve Steps and these excerpts in connection with
programs and activities which are patterned after AA, but which address other
problems, or in any other non-AA context, does not imply otherwise.

To those dually disordered individuals who have lost family, friends, and faith because of their dual disorders; to those of us who have stood by helplessly as we watched our loved ones destroyed by their dual diseases; and for my brother Tom, who took his own life, desperate and alone, because of his dual diseases. May they find peace of mind for their restless spirits in the next dimension, a gift that this life could not provide them.

K. E.

For family, friends, and all others who have helped

J. M. S.

About the Authors

Katie Evans, PhD, NCACII, has a PhD in clinical psychology and is an Oregon Board Certified alcohol and drug counselor and a nationally credited alcohol and drug counselor. She is currently CEO and Treatment Coordinator at the Evans & Sullivan Clinic, where she works with both adults and adolescents who have coexisting substance abuse and psychological problems. Dr. Evans specializes in counseling survivors of abuse who are chemically dependent. Over the past 20 years, Dr. Evans has worked with individuals who have psychological and chemical use problems, as well as with their families. In addition to working as a therapist, she has served as the clinical director for several inpatient as well as outpatient programs servicing both adults and teenagers. She is also an active consultant to numerous agencies and treatment centers in the United States and Europe and is on the faculty of Portland State University. An author of many articles and pamphlets on various mental health services and substance abuse recovery topics, Dr. Evans has coauthored several books with J. Michael Sullivan, including the first edition of *Dual Diagnosis, Step Study Counseling with the Dual Disordered Client, Recovering from Post-Traumatic Stress Disorder and Addiction,* and *Treating Addicted Survivors of Trauma.* Dr. Evans also conducts workshops and seminars nationally and internationally on a variety of mental health and recovery-related topics.

J. Michael Sullivan, PhD, is a licensed clinical psychologist and has practiced in a number of inpatient and outpatient settings, both public and private. For the past 15 years, Dr. Sullivan has specialized in the treatment of persons suffering from dual disorders. With Katie Evans, he opened the Evans & Sullivan Clinic, a dual diagnosis outpatient treatment program, and serves as its clinical director. Dr. Sullivan also provides supervision as well as direct clinical services to adults and adolescents. With Katie Evans, he has cowritten numerous books, articles, and client materials dealing with the assessment and treatment of dual disorders, including the first edition of *Dual Diagnosis* and *Treating Addicted*

Survivors of Trauma. Other publications include the series of client pamphlets, *Understanding Your Dual Diagnosis.* Dr. Sullivan has also given workshops on dual diagnosis, both on his own and with Dr. Evans, in the United States and abroad, and has served as a consultant to various dual diagnosis programs and task forces.

Preface

Welcome to the second edition of *Dual Diagnosis: Counseling the Mentally Ill Substance Abuser.*

How can we provide quality services for individuals with dual diagnoses? Numerous developments in the field in general and in our own experience have provided the context and stimulus for this second edition. Managed health care and its impact on the provision of services is arguably the most important of these developments during the past 10 years. Gone are the days of routinely and readily admitting clients to chemical dependency programs for 28 days or to psychiatric units for a month or more. Instead, care has shifted to outpatient settings, often for longer periods of time. Even detoxification is now at times an outpatient procedure. Case managers for third-party payers demand clear and detailed clinical justification for any proposed treatment plan and do so throughout treatment. Third-party payers have increased their demands that providers be suitably credentialed and trained in treatments with empirically demonstrated effectiveness. Not even the public sector has been immune to these changes. Now, more than ever, providers need both breadth and depth of expertise and must be prepared to treat very ill and troubled clients in an outpatient setting.

Since we wrote the first edition, our own clinical practice has shifted from mainly an inpatient to an outpatient one, with the establishment of our own outpatient clinic. We see a somewhat different mix of clients and see them over a longer period of time. Among other things, these changes have increased our appreciation of the difference between acute and long-term care and the importance of motivation and of relapse–prevention issues. We have enhanced experience applying the Twelve Steps with dually disordered individuals. We have written an entire book on posttraumatic stress disorder and addiction (*Treating Addicted Survivors of Trauma*; Evans & Sullivan, 1995) that deepened our understanding of dual disorder treatment in general. We have presented workshops at many conferences in the United States and abroad, and have learned from other presenters and our audiences. Katie Evans is now "Doctor" Evans, with the completion of her doctorate in clinical psychology.

As in the first edition, in this volume we use 12-step recovery concepts as the main framework for integrating substance use disorder and mental health treatments. We have, however, made some important changes even as we have maintained the general framework, theoretical stance, and tone of the book. These changes include the following:

1. Updating the discussion of the issues that clients with dual diagnoses present, with a new commentary on managed health care.
2. Making current our discussion of treatment interventions for both substance use and mental health disorders.
3. Using concepts and terminology of the fourth edition of the *Diagnostic and Statistical Manual of Mental Disorders* (DSM-IV).
4. Increasing the discussion of ways to integrate 12-step concepts into actual sessions with clients and to apply them to both disorders.
5. Deleting the section on passive–aggressive clients, a move consistent with DSM-IV changes.
6. Combining the sections on schizophrenia and organic mental disorders in one chapter because of similarities in therapeutic interventions.
7. Adding a section on the treatment of trauma-based disorders with addicted female adolescents.
8. Incorporating relapse prevention issues into the sections on each disorder rather than in a separate section.
9. Enhancing the discussion of motivating clients.

We have made every effort to present the most recent literature and research available in the area of dual diagnosis treatment as of this writing. However, the treatment suggestions here are from our own clinical experiences and are based on what has worked for the hundreds of clients we have treated over the past 11 years since our original writing. Writing this book is an opportunity for us to introduce readers to dual diagnosis treatment and to offer practical therapeutic approaches, as well as provide ways for more seasoned practitioners to enhance their skills.

Acknowledgments

We would like to thank our families, who supported us during the writing of this updated edition. We are also grateful to The Guilford Press for its support of our efforts; to Rick Ries, MD, who has supported our work and encouraged us to stay current in research while we work as full-time clinicians; and to Stanton Samenow, PhD, who gave us permission to use his material on thinking errors. We share a deep appreciation for our long-standing collaboration. Through our differences in background and life experiences, we continue to share with our clients and you, the reader, a well-balanced perspective for working with the dually disordered population. We wish to thank our clients, from whom we have learned much. Most importantly, we want to thank the mentors in our academic, professional, and personal lives who gave us the motivation, support, and spiritual guidance that has continued to illuminate our path. We hope that this writing helps you shine a bit of brightness and hope into the dark corners of despair in which many dually diagnosed individuals dwell. Shine your light!

Contents

CHAPTER 1

The Nature of the Problem

One drink is too many and a thousand is never enough.
—ALCOHOLICS ANONYMOUS

DOUBLE TROUBLE
Definition of Dual Diagnosis

How can we assess and treat clients who present with both a substance abuse or dependence problem and a coexisting psychiatric disorder? The term "dual diagnosis" is a general designation used to describe those individuals who suffer from comorbid substance abuse/dependence as well as a psychotic, affective, behavioral, or severe personality disorder (Lehman, 1996). Persons with such double disorders often pose a "double" treatment challenge.

Epidemiology

Individuals with a psychiatric disorder are at increased risk for having a comorbid substance abuse disorder, and vice versa. The Epidemiologic Catchment Area (ECA) Study found that 29% of all persons with mental disorders have met the criteria for a substance abuse disorder at some time in their past and that suffering from a mental disorder increased the odds of having a substance use disorder by 2.7 times (Regier et al., 1990). Some 37 percent of those with an alcohol disorder had a comorbid disorder. Slightly more than half (53%) of those with a substance use disorder involving chemicals other than alcohol also had a comorbid mental disorder. In treatment settings (including both chemical dependence and mental health settings) nearly 20 percent of persons suffering from a mental disorder met the criteria for a substance use disorder during the preceding 6 months. Fifty-five percent of individuals with alcohol disorders had a coexisting mental disorder within the preceding 6 months, and those with drug disorders other than alcohol had a rate of 64%.

The National Comorbidity Survey also found not only a heightened risk of drug use disorders among those with alcohol disorders but also a higher risk of alcohol use disorders being associated with comorbid psychiatric disorders (Kessler et al., 1997). This association held whether the alcohol use disorder or the psychiatric disorder was reported as occurring first, and was especially true for women.

Diagnostic and Treatment Difficulties

Individuals abusing or dependent on drugs can develop symptoms similar to those seen in many psychiatric disorders (Margolis & Zweben, 1998), including psychotic symptoms, depression, anxiety, mood swings, and isolation and social withdrawal, as well as erratic, hostile, or self-centered relationships and criminal behavior. Alcoholics, for example, demonstrate a high prevalence of both transient, temporarily persistent, anxiety and panic symptoms in early recovery, but only 6–7% (still twice the rate of the general population, however) demonstrate chronic anxiety disorders (Schuckit & Hesselbrock, 1994).

Several questions, then, face the evaluator assessing clients. Are this person's problems caused mainly by the chemicals or the psychiatric disorder—or both? Is there misuse, abuse, or dependence? Will the client be served better in a mental health setting or in a chemical dependency program—or does he/she need a special dual diagnosis program? When the managed health care coordinator asks which diagnosis is primary, what is the answer?

Engaging persons with dual diagnoses in treatment can also be especially difficult. Alcoholics and addicts often do not admit to others or themselves that they have a problem with substances and, instead, minimize or rationalize their use and associated problems. Psychiatric clients also often deny their disorders. Dual clients are often doubly in denial and doubly difficult to enlist into treatment (Levy, 1993; Osher & Kofoed, 1989).

Many dually diagnosed persons are, in addition, unable to comply with treatment or to benefit from standard interventions because of the complications of both illnesses. Understanding lectures on the negative effects of drugs is difficult for those people with impaired concentration. For example, individuals with a history of alcohol dependence, especially those early in recovery and those who are older, show significant cognitive impairments (Goldman, 1990). Individuals with major depression also have significant cognitive deficits (Elliott, Sahakian, McKay, Robbins, & Paykel, 1996). The two together create double the difficulties in thinking and learning.

What about the person suffering from both the disease of addiction and a major mental illness? Attending self-help groups may be challenging for persons who are seriously depressed and find it difficult to get out of bed, or for persons who are paranoid and are convinced others are talking about them (e.g., Morgenstern, Lavbouvie, McCrady, Kahler, & Frey, 1997). For someone who suffers from anxiety and mood disorders, drinking even moderately will interfere with the effectiveness of prescribed medication (Castenada, Sussman, Westreich, Levy, & O'Malley, 1996). Helping clients with dual disorders accept the difference between chemicals of abuse and medications with therapeutic impact can be tricky. Intense and demanding confrontations of the sort often used with persons who are just alcoholic or addicted will sometimes increase the psychotic symptoms or suicidal ideation of dually diagnosed persons.

Conflicts in Philosophy and the Stigma of These Illnesses

Philosophical conflicts and a fragmented service system continue to compound the difficulties facing providers, persons with dual disorders, and their families. Society has tended to view alcoholism and addiction as moral and legal issues. Individuals with chemical use difficulties are seen as bad people who lack willpower and suffer from a defective character. The "war on drugs" and the emphasis on fines and imprisonment reflect this point of view. Similarly, society has historically tended to view many mental disorders as the result of poor motivation or a weak character. The individual who suffers from either a substance disorder or a psychiatric disorder faces the stigma and shame associated with his/her illness and often receives advice that says "Snap out of it!" Both individuals suffering from dual disorders and their families may still operate from a shamed-based model in which they feel "bad" or "guilty" for both their addictions and their mental disorders. The legal and moral models compound the shame and increase the likelihood that dually disordered clients and their families will not seek treatment.

Many mental health professionals are reluctant to treat alcoholics and addicts, even those with a coexisting psychiatric disorder. This reluctance may stem from their own failures and frustrations in treating those actively addicted through psychotherapy approaches. We have heard many fine therapists speak with despair about their clients relapsing on alcohol or other drugs, lying, defending their right to use chemicals, and carrying out all the negative behaviors associated with the addictive disease process. Therapists are left feeling ineffective, or they begin to view addicted individuals as resistant to traditional mental health approaches or as unlikely to benefit from treatment so long as they con-

tinue to use substances. At the same time, chemical dependency counselors often either refuse to treat those with comorbid mental health
problems or find themselves dealing with problems well beyond their
scope of training.

Treatment Systems Lack Integration

Programs and staff for the treatment of psychiatric and chemical dependency disorders are typically separate or, at best, have a psychiatric consultant, or one drug/alcohol expert, depending on the setting. Few professionals have the necessary cross-training to effectively integrate the
synergistic treatments needed for this special population. Many state and
county governments have separate departments for mental health and
for addiction. This separation, while done to preserve the integrity of
both fields, makes it doubly difficult to enact needed legislative changes
to enable the mentally ill addict to obtain services from one or both systems. Attempts to utilize both systems at once for treatment also often
leave consumers confused due to the differences in the philosophical
approaches of two different agencies and overwhelmed at managing different sets of appointments, counselors, and so forth.

Separate training programs for psychologists, social workers, and
addiction counselors are still the norm. Thus, the opportunities to learn
from one another get lost in the academic shuffle. The insistence on
licensure for all providers has left many addiction counselors who are
"certified" but not "licensed" out of the loop for the treatment of many
addicted clients. These counselors' expertise, in addition to being un-
available to clients, is threatened with extinction unless the counselors
can be grandfathered into licensure or can pursue the graduate degrees
that make licensure a possibility.

Funding sources make it difficult to provide effective integrated
treatment for the dually disordered person. Our experience is that many
public and private funding sources still provide widely disparate benefit
levels for the two sets of disorders, forcing clinicians to decide which of
the two main disorders is "primary."

Managed health care has added another layer of administration.
Obtaining treatment authorization from many managed health care
plans tends to focus on treatment only of acute symptoms. Brief strategic treatment interventions effective in the merely neurotic are seen
as a beneficial option for the dually disordered client. Many providers
who want to treat the dually disordered person in a comprehensive way
are faced with moral, ethical, and financial dilemmas regarding what
is in the client's best interest, given the limited availability of treatment
funding.

Fragmented Treatment

Federal and state agencies have earmarked money to be used to provide assessment and treatment services to indigent adults and youth. Each state, county, and community agency utilizes these funds to meet the identified need in its area. When mentally ill clients present themselves at the community alcohol program for assessment and treatment, several problems may arise.

An intoxicated individual reporting hearing voices at the time of an assessment poses difficulties in discriminating whether he/she is experiencing drug- or alcohol-induced psychosis or suffering from an independent psychotic disorder. To determine whether a psychiatric hospital or a detox center is the best setting for stabilization, one needs a good psychiatric and chemical dependency history of the individual. Unfortunately, since psychotic persons usually exhibit poor reality testing and there may be a lack of collateral contacts, a clear and accurate history may be difficult to obtain. To make matters even worse, denial is likely to further distort the picture.

If the person seeks help first in an alcohol and drug setting, the chemical dependency counselor's logical course might be to refer or admit the individual to a detox center, to allow for a sober assessment of the individual. Due to the common symptom of alcoholic hallucinosis, such a referral with the focus on sobriety is a logical one. Shortly into detox, it may become clear that the client's problems are more complicated than usually seen with a chemically induced psychosis. The detoxifying patient may exhibit strange, psychotic, and/or somewhat threatening behavior. The detox center, not staffed or equipped to manage such symptoms, may end up transferring the client to an acute psychiatric hospital. However, the hospital, while stabilizing the client, may not address the substance use disorder or may have difficulty finding a treatment program in the community that will enroll the client. Mental health centers often exclude persons with substance abuse, and chemical dependence centers often rule out those with a history of serious psychiatric problems. The client then falls through the cracks.

The Legal System Isn't a Treatment System

Those providers who work in the criminal justice system know the relationship between substance abuse and criminal activity. The use of illegal drugs in and of itself is a criminal offense in most states. It is highly unlikely that the average dually diagnosed client surviving on a limited income can afford frequent consumption of chemicals. Therefore, dually diagnosed individuals often do not pay their bills. If they don't pay their rent, for example, they end up in an eviction proceeding with the landlord and ultimately become homeless; alternatively, they may try to support their habit through dealing drugs, prostitution, or other illegal activities.

Depending on the nature of the psychiatric illness and the types of drugs these persons abuse, they may find themselves arrested on a number of different charges. Drunk and disorderly conduct, shoplifting, drug trafficking, solicitation, and theft are not altogether uncommon aspects of the life of the dually disordered person. For the antisocial addict, burglary and theft are the most common ways for the drug abuser to obtain money. For the psychiatrically impaired individual with psychotic and disorganized thinking, the ability to mastermind a serious crime or consistently engage in criminal activity without getting caught can be an extremely tenuous proposition. Closing state hospitals en masse has also led to the rapid proliferation of homeless persons who often have dual diagnoses and who are commonly arrrested for a variety of reasons.

Once arrested, individuals enter the criminal justice system. The court system is not designed to serve as a treatment alternative for the mentally ill. While they are held in jail, it may quickly become obvious that they need medical assistance. Either a single overworked nurse attempts to provide care, or individuals are transferred to another facility, one most like not designed to handle clients with dual disorders. After stabilization of the acute crisis, the individuals are either immediately returned to jail or released. Or, following arraignment, persons are released pending a hearing and, again, return to the community untreated. No treatment or rehabilitation has taken place.

Youth at Risk

In the case of adolescents, the issue of dual disorders presents itself in a slightly different light. Child protective services experts have shared with us that in the vast majority of child abuse cases the perpetrator was abusing drugs or alcohol. An environment in which abuse of chemicals and violence are present is a breeding ground for emotional and psychological problems in children. Social workers working in the area of child protective services who identify parental substance abuse as a problem have no authority to require parents to seek help. The judicial authority granted child protective service workers is through the juvenile court system, which has legal authority only over children.

Recent shootings at various schools around the country have brought to light the perilous mental health of some of our youth. Rates of major depression and suicide among youth have been increasing dramatically (Anthony, Warner, & Kessler, 1994). Surveys show that the rates of drug use, after dropping during the early 1990s, are now increasing, even among youth in the junior high/middle school (Grant & Pickering, 1996). As school funding levels have slipped, the availability of counselors and other resources for children in trouble has substantially decreased. Educators have little to no training in this area and are already burdened with multiple duties. Our clinical experience attests that many of our troubled young people have dual disorders. However, the resources are not available to help them.

Financial Cost and Managed Health Care

During the late 1980s businesses became alarmed at the skyrocketing cost of insurance premiums, and economists voiced chagrin over the increasing amounts of the gross national product dedicated to health expenditures. Managed health care has attempted to control costs by introducing a mix of measures, including collective bargaining with providers to enforce price reductions and freezes, precertification and concurrent review of treatment, and an emphasis on adhering strictly to the criterion of paying only for "medically necessary" treatments.

Substance dependence is a chronic illness (as are many mental disorders), requiring ongoing treatment for many months, if not years. Managed health care reviewers, however, often will allow treatment only if symptoms are "acute" and will normally disallow coverage for ongoing maintenance treatment. Being discharged prematurely from treatment often leads to a relapse in both comorbid illnesses.

Treatment centers have closed and provider incomes have fallen because of the limited funding available for addiction services. Finding sufficient staff with expertise in both mental health and chemical dependence has always been tricky. But this has become increasingly difficult with the decreasing ability to adequately compensate individuals for enhancing their skills and working with a challenging treatment population.

Cost to Clients and Families

Family members and relatives of the dually diagnosed person will often find themselves depleted emotionally and financially. They may find that they are moving from crisis to crisis, stretching thin the patience and tolerance of even the most supportive family. The individual with a dual diagnosis can become violent and threatening toward family members. This kind of behavior can force the family to shut out the person in order to protect themselves. Their attempts to find adequate care for their loved one are often met with limited coverage from private health plans. Public funding is often scarce and limited to only low-income families.

Stricken by the disease of chemical dependency and suffering from a psychiatric disorder, the individual with dual disorders is not well armed to deal with systems conflicts. Persons enter expensive private psychiatric hospitals or seek counseling from private practitioners, where treatment professionals may not address their substance abuse problems. The same persons enter private chemical dependency programs where their mental health issues may be put on hold until sobriety is established. However, the dually diagnosed person has a difficult time attaining sobriety for any length of time without getting help for the coexisting psychiatric problems. Each unsuccessful treatment experience adds to the person's confusion and feelings of worthlessness. With neither illness adequately treated, the client moves ever closer to such self-defeating settings as jail, permanent or semipermanent institutionalization, or a health-related hastened death.

A COMPOSITE CASE EXAMPLE: "TIM"

Tim, an 18-year-old male suffering from schizophrenia, was receiving voluntary treatment through an outpatient community mental health center. He was being given Prolixin shots, as he had previously been noncompliant with oral medications. His case manager had become concerned that Tim might be experimenting with marijuana.

Tim was starting to miss appointments, and his parents reported that he was socializing with a peer group of delinquent adolescents in the neighborhood. When Tim did appear for an appointment, he was moody, avoidant, and displayed an increasingly negative attitude toward the case manager. In response the case manager scheduled a meeting with both Tim and his parents, but Tim again missed the appointment. When Tim's parents met with the counselor, they acknowledged that they had once found Tim smoking marijuana in his room—but they thought it a purely transitory experience and were not seriously alarmed. The case manager ended up referring Tim to an outpatient chemical dependency program for an evaluation, but Tim again did not show up for the appointment. When the case manager contacted Tim's parents to reschedule, they informed the case manager that they would be taking Tim to another clinic for his medication and requested that the case manager close Tim's file.

Two weeks following the closure of his case, Tim was arrested by police. High on drugs and off his medication, he had stolen a city bus and proceeded to smash it into two parked cars and a police vehicle before apprehension. Tim was taken to the county jail, where he had to be placed into five-point restraints because of his psychosis and violent behavior. Fortunately for Tim, his family had financial resources and actively involved themselves in arranging treatment for him. He was transferred from jail to an acute psychiatric hospital, where a dual diagnosis unit was better able to assess and meet Tim's clinical needs. Tim was treated as an inpatient for 3 weeks. By the time he was transferred from the hospital to an outpatient dual diagnosis program, Tim was able to admit consciously that he suffered from addiction and a mental illness.

CONCLUSION

Tim's case illustrates several issues, chief among them the need to take both disorders—the mental illness and the addictive behavior—seriously. It also illustrates the special challenges that dual diagnosis treatment poses for clients, families, and providers. And the composite case study illustrates one other thing, namely, that *successful treatment is possible.* Succeeding chapters in this volume provide some specific solutions to some of the problems raised in this chapter, with an emphasis on clinical aspects of the dually diagnosed individual's situation.

CHAPTER 2

Models of Treatment

> One psychiatrist I saw said that I should take Valium
> instead of drinking. I guess he thought I suffered from a
> Valium deficiency.
> —MEMBER OF ALCOHOLICS ANONYMOUS

In this chapter we will outline some commonly used treatment approaches for substance dependence and for mental health disorders, emphasizing issues that have an impact on decisions about dual diagnosis treatment. We will examine interventions for clients with dual diagnoses and present the available outcome data for these interventions.

MODELS OF SUBSTANCE DEPENDENCE TREATMENT

The majority of treatment professionals subscribes to the biopsychosocial model of addiction. This model posits that there is not only an inherited and an induced biological component to addictive disorders but also psychological–behavioral and social–cultural factors that have a role in the cause, course, and outcome of substance dependence. During the past decade a consensus has also evolved that, while there is no one universally and uniquely effective approach for curing substance dependence, treatments specifically targeting substance use are demonstrably efficacious (e.g., McLellan et al., 1994). While there are possible pitfalls in integrating addiction treatment models (McCrady, 1994), treatment programs are typically eclectic and manage successfully to blend compatible interventions without regard to theoretical purity. The standard set of interventions typically includes arrangements for detoxification, education and skills-building classes, group therapy, family involvement, relapse prevention activities, and referral to 12-step programs.

Three different paradigms of addiction and its treatment are most influential (Margolis & Zweben, 1998; McCrady, 1994). One paradigm holds that the person's problematic chemical involvement is really a symptom of, or a response to, a psychiatric disturbance or a family dysfunction. There are several variants on this theme. One derives from a psychoanalytic–developmental perspective (Khantzian, 1997). Persons with substance use disorders had maladaptive parenting that left them with problems in tolerating negative feelings, taking care of themselves, having good self-esteem, and developing intimate relationships. These persons then use chemicals to self-medicate and cope with the problems such deficits cause. Even if not due to faulty development, the self-medication hypothesis holds that the alcoholic or addicted person abuses chemicals in a well-meaning but problem-producing attempt to alleviate psychic pain and manage the symptoms of the "underlying" mental, emotional, or behavioral problem. Another variant assumes that the alcoholic or addicted individual is really responding to marital conflict or other family dysfunctions (McCrady & Epstein, 1996). The implication of this symptom-of-something-else notion is straightforward: successfully treat the underlying problem, and clients will moderate or end the problematic substance use.

Other paradigms focus on the chemical use and dependency as a problem in its own right. Learning theory models constitute one of these paradigms. Classical (Pavlovian) conditioning, where environmental or internal cues become associated with use, helps to explain cravings. Operant conditioning explains how the immediate rewards of chemicals, including the positive reinforcement of euphoria and negative reinforcement of relief from cravings and anxiety, influence behavior more than the longer-term negative consequences of substance abuse and addiction. Cognitive-behavioral models look at the importance of thoughts and emotions in influencing behavior and emphasize the learning of skills to enhance self-efficacy in managing chemical misuse habits.

These models have led to treatment approaches such as aversive conditioning, where the sight, smell, and taste of alcohol is paired with a noxious stimulus such as an electric shock or chemically induced vomiting, or cue exposure treatments, where experimenters have addicts look at and touch drug paraphernalia without the reinforcement of drug use (Childress, Hole, Ehrman, & Robbins, 1993). Prescribing Antabuse (disulfiram) to produce an aversive reaction to any alcohol intake or Trexan (naltrexone) to block the effects of opiates are other examples of intervention designed to change the operant contingencies associated with chemical use. The term "relapse prevention" refers to a set of cognitive-behavioral interventions that are widely used in treatment. Relapse prevention has two general strategies (Annis & Davis, 1989; Gorski, 1989). The first is to help clients become aware of cues and patterns of thinking, feeling, and behaving that lead to chemical use through discussion, questionnaires, and self-monitoring homework assignments. The second is to enhance clients' coping skills by helping them make plans to handle triggers, learn skills to handle negative feelings such as progressive muscular relaxation, and change dysfunctional thinking patterns through a technique such as writing down counterarguments.

One widely used paradigm views addiction as a chronic disease. Alcoholism (and, by extension, any drug dependence) is a biologically based disorder in which environmental factors activate a genetic predisposition (Leshner, 1997; Begleiter & Kissin, 1995; Tarter & Vanyukov, 1994). Prolonged use of chemicals modifies neurotransmitter and neuropeptide systems of the brain involved in the regulation of primary drive states to create chemical-use drive states similar to those involving thirst, hunger, and sex (Miller & Chappell, 1991). Long-lasting brain changes involve such phenomena as brain metabolic activity, neuron membrane and synaptic function, gene expression, and reactions to environmental cues (Christie & Mitchell, 2000). Furthermore, alcoholism has specific diagnostic signs and symptoms and a predictable course. Interventions have the goals of abstinence or reduction in use, reduction in the frequency and severity of relapse, and improvement in functioning (e.g., Kinney, 1996). Such interventions might include detoxification if needed. As with other chronic illnesses such as diabetes, educating clients about the signs and symptoms of their illness and the steps necessary for managing it is crucial. Developing a long-term management plan and monitoring compliance carefully are both important. The plan may include the use of dietary supplements, exercise, regular check-ins with treatment personal, and perhaps the use of such medications as naltrexone or disulfiram (O'Brien, 1996). Referral to support groups, most usually 12-step programs, is also a crucial part of this plan, as is specific relapse prevention activities. Educating and involving family members is an important part of treatment, as well. Psychosocial habilitation programs focusing on such things as vocational counseling address other concomitants of the disease.

In the next section we will review in more detail the variant on the disease paradigm known as the recovery model, which has been very influential, not just in general, but also on our own thinking about dual diagnosis treatment. Also, many mental health professionals are not familiar with the details of 12-step programs, and at least some familiarity is necessary for understanding the remainder of this volume and for making client referrals to 12-step programs.

THE RECOVERY MODEL

The recovery model views chemical dependency as a disease. This disease is chronic (it does not go away), it is progressive (it worsens with time), and it is likely to be ultimately fatal (if not arrested through abstinence). And, as with many other diseases such as hypertension or diabetes, relapses are frequent and common and thus to be expected.

The American Medical Association has maintained for decades that substance dependence is a disease. Adoption and twin studies, genetic breeding and brain physiology studies of animals, and natural history studies of alcoholics all support this point of view (Margolis & Zweeben, 1998; Kinney, 1996). Nevertheless, the general public and even many professionals have difficulty in believing or understanding how chemical dependency can be a disease.

Probably the most difficult aspect for many to accept about the disease paradigm is not the notion that alcohol dependence has a genetic component, a set of defining symptoms, or a predictable course, but rather the idea that the alcoholic and addict truly do not have a choice—that they have lost control of their drinking and using. Labeling them as sick might seem to absolve the alcoholic and addict of responsibility. The behavior of an alcoholic or addict can be so distasteful and painful to those around him/her that the resulting emotions can obstruct efforts aimed at caring for a sick friend. Given the plethora of negative emotions and difficult experiences associated with alcoholics and addicts, people tend to see these individuals as bad instead of sick. It is for precisely this reason that an approach that treats chemically dependent people as *sick people getting well rather than bad people getting good* is useful.

The disease process recovery model provides a safe and supportive treatment framework free of moralizing and condemnation. The recovery model assists the chemically dependent person in looking at his/her old bad behavior and reframing it as sick behavior. Relapse in this context is not a failing on the part of the client (or the treatment provider!). Slogans such as "one day at a time" and "easy does it" enable the alcoholic to see that he/she is now on a journey, a journey of recovery. Responsibility lies not in having the disease but in successfully implementing a recovery program.

The recovery model assumes that an alcoholic is never fully recovered, but rather always in the process of recovery. The disease is *chronic.* In order for one to stay on the journey of recovery, certain events must occur. To begin the journey the alcoholic or addict must first identify him/herself as an alcoholic or addict. A refusal to accept that one suf-

fers from the disease of chemical dependency only increases the likelihood that drinking and drug-abusing behavior will resume. Addicts
need to learn about the signs and symptoms of their disease as part of
this process and to accept in their own heart that they suffer from this
disease.

In addition, information regarding damage done to body, mind, and
spirit (as well as to family members) needs to be provided to assist the
person in understanding that chemical dependency is dangerous and
chronic. The disease lurks in wait for that person to take the first pill,
fix, or drink. Some sort of abstinence (even if interrupted by occasional
relapses) is mandatory before any substantial recovery can begin. The
chemically dependent person must also understand that use of any mood-
altering chemicals will most likely lead to addiction to a new drug or a
return to old patterns of addiction.

The alcoholic or addict must also learn about cross-tolerance and
addiction. One of the features of alcoholism is *metabolic tolerance,* which
refers to the process by which the body adapts to the presence of alcohol. As this process occurs, the body learns to tolerate larger and larger
doses of alcohol without experiencing the effects normally associated with
increased use. The symptom of tolerance is one way of distinguishing a
social drinker from an alcoholic. The middle-stage alcoholic can frequently drink everyone under the table while showing only mild signs of
intoxication. For the person who has this metabolic adaptation, the use
of any central nervous system depressant will produce the same effects;
that is, the normally prescribed dosage of Valium, Xanax, Dalmane, or
other sedative-type drugs will have only minimal effect on the alcoholic.
We have been told by recovering alcoholics who were in car wrecks or
had surgery that they had difficulty in becoming sedated or anesthetized
because of this phenomenon.

Because alcohol is a depressant drug like tranquilizers and sedatives, it is imperative that recovering alcoholics steer clear of all mood-
altering drugs in attempts to protect their sobriety. It is not uncommon
to hear recovering alcoholics discuss how they were prescribed Xanax
for a panic disorder, or used other chemicals when not drinking, only
to find that they now had become addicted to these drugs. This phenomenon is known as *cross-addiction.* In our experience alcoholics and addicts
will also often switch their drug of choice to other classes of chemicals
outside the depressant category and establish new addictions to other
chemicals. Priming doses of any drugs can trigger drug cravings through
activation of the mesolimbic dopamine system (Self, 1998; Self & Nestler,
1998).

It is important to remember that chemical dependency is a *disease.*
Physiologically, the addict's body processes and metabolizes all chemi-

cals differently than in nonaddicted persons. Therefore, a safe and successful recovery program must be based on abstinence from *all* mood-altering chemicals. Acceptance of and belief that one suffers from a disease is paramount, since no true recovery can begin without this belief. It is important to remember that addiction is a *primary* urge, taking precedence over relationships, money, food, and shelter. One doesn't wake up one morning and say to oneself, Gee, today I think I'll stop doing the one thing that is most important to my life. Not unless there is a good reason! Acceptance that the disease of addiction is chronic, progressive, and often fatal can help a client realistically look at his/her drinking and using behavior. Alcoholics Anonymous states point-blank that jails, institutions, and death await the practicing addict.

In addition to education about the disease and its effects, peer support as well as peer confrontation are important. Using chemicals leads addicts to develop a skewed sense of themselves and their relationship to the world. Peers can point out unrealistic views of self and world and can assist the addict in gaining needed emotional growth—growth hitherto stunted by the use of drugs and alcohol.

Skills-building activities and other psychosocial therapies are extremely important. The disease of addiction, among other things, prevents the individual from learning social and other coping skills. Thus, assertiveness training and stress management can be an excellent start, as is family counseling. Abstinence is the start of recovery, but more is needed.

Discussion of the recovery model would be incomplete without a discussion of Alcoholics Anonymous (AA) and the Twelve Steps, especially AA's focus on spirituality. While AA is not a treatment program, the major goal of treatment from within the recovery paradigm is to teach the patient not to rely on the therapist ultimately but to actively work the Twelve Steps of AA and to use the AA fellowship and its resources (meetings, sponsorship, hotline, social events, and so forth) to the maximum.

THE TWELVE STEPS OF AA*

Listed below are the steps of AA and an explanation of the meaning of the steps (Alcoholics Anonymous, 1976). They are suggestive only. Dr. Bob and Bill W., the founders of AA, well understood the willful nature of the alcoholic.

---

*The Twelve Steps reprinted with permission of Alcoholics Anonymous World Services, Inc. AA is a program of recovery from alcoholism only. There are programs patterned after AA that address other problems of addiction and substance abuse.

1. We admitted we were powerless over alcohol; that our lives had become unmanageable. Those who have had experience with Step 1 understand the paradox of this step: only by admitting to powerlessness does the individual become empowered to make healthy choices for him/herself. Most chemically dependent people have made countless but fruitless attempts to control their alcohol and drug use and be solely a social drinker or user. They have also attempted to control and mitigate the negative consequences of their chemical use. Identifying that, in spite of all their efforts to control the uncontrollable, they eventually lose control provides the foundation on which chemically dependent persons can build their recovery. The alcoholic or addict must truly believe that his/her use of chemicals and the consequences of their use point to a disease process that he/she is powerless to control. The surrender of all this control releases the alcoholic/addict from a heavy burden. By labeling themselves as recovering addicts and alcoholics, these people begin to accept that they suffer from a disease that is chronic, progressive, fatal, and without a cure. Only remission is possible, at best, and this can be achieved only through abstinence. The insight, or acceptance, that a problem exists is the goal of this first step. Contemplation of the negative consequences of chemical use also enhances motivation to change.

2. Came to believe that a power greater than ourselves could restore us to sanity. Step 2 establishes hope and faith in an individual whose life has in recent times greatly lacked either commodity. The mention of a power greater than ourselves helps the alcoholic/addict to begin looking for help from others, which is a decidedly different strategy from the leave-me-alone, I'll-do-it-myself attitude so common in the chemically dependent person. The insanity alluded to in this step attempts to begin to address what is sometimes referred to as "stinkin' thinkin'." This is the denial and antisocial, self-centered world view of the practicing alcoholic, which, once identified, is slowly chipped away through continual and ongoing involvement in working the Twelve Steps or participating in similar 12-step programs. Often insanity is defined as repeating the same behavior and yet expecting different results. Consequently, another goal of this step is to assist individuals in identifying the unhelpful solutions that they have previously tried as preparation for choosing more helpful ones.

3. Made a decision to turn our will and our lives over to the care of God, as we understood Him. Step 3 helps the alcoholic to learn to turn over, or let go of, problems or worry over which the alcoholic has no control. Obsessive worry and fear tend to paralyze the alcoholic and make clear thinking and good problem solving extremely difficult. In order to turn something over, it is necessary to have a concept of who or what you are going to turn it over to. This step clearly invokes, the aid of "God, *as we understood Him*—"leaving open a variety of choices for who or what God is to the chemically dependent person as an individual. Many individuals raised in the Christian tradition choose the God of their childhood upbringing. Those who are perhaps rebelling from it establish their own personal concept of a higher power. Many alcoholics/addicts choose their AA or Narcotics Anonymous (NA) group as a collective higher power. Who or what the higher power is must always be the choice of the individual. AA and NA are spiritual programs, not organized religion. They do not require a belief in a prescribed higher power. This step also emphasizes the positive action of committing to doing things someone else's way, someone with a higher wisdom.

4. Made a searching and fearless moral inventory of ourselves. The moral inventory described in this step is the process by which alcoholics can become relieved of their heavy burden of anger, resentment, fear, and guilt. A written inventory whereby the alcoholic or addict takes a look at how he/she was often the maker of his/her own problems is generally the best. This spiritual, emotional, and psychological housecleaning lightens the emotional load of the alcoholic or addict. This step also attempts to help the person develop an honest, realistic picture of him/herself and is analogous to many of the processes that occur in longer-term psychotherapy.

5. Admitted to God, to ourselves, and to another human being the exact nature of our wrongs. In this step the chemically dependent person discusses the content of Step 4 with another person as well as with the higher power. By freely discussing the hidden burden, the power of old secrets to create shame is dissolved, and open, honest communication is made possible. As has often been said, confession is good for the soul.

6. Were entirely ready to have God remove all these defects of character. This step readies the chemically dependent person for further change. Realizing where he/she erred in the past makes the alcoholic ready to seek help from other places, including a higher power. Part of this process entails the dissolution of the perverse narcissistic investment persons often have in their own negative characteristics. To change these destructive patterns is the goal of Step 6.

7. Humbly asked Him to remove our shortcomings. This step is the beginning of humility and true self-esteem. Bragging, grandiose ways of relating to the world are exchanged for humility and the beginnings of peace of mind.

8. Made a list of all persons we had harmed, and became willing to make amends to them all. Growing spiritually, the alcoholic becomes very aware of how the alcoholic and addictive behavior was hurtful not only to him/herself but to others. In this step the alcoholic makes a list of all those people he or she has harmed and is now willing to try to make amends to and apologize to for previous behavior.

9. Made direct amends to such people wherever possible, except when to do so would injure them or others. In this step the alcoholic makes direct amends and apologizes to those individuals wronged previously by his or her destructive behavior. Through this process the alcoholic/addict continues to build humility and gains peace of mind by cleaning up the wreckage of the past.

10. Continued to take personal inventory, and when we were wrong promptly admitted it. This is a maintenance step. By keeping a clean house through working an honest program, the alcoholic keeps from falling into old behaviors that can lead to relapse back into drinking and using behavior.

11. Sought through prayer and meditation to improve our conscious contact with God **as we understood Him,** *praying only for knowledge of His will for us and the power to carry that out.* The alcoholic now begins more fully to comprehend spirituality. He or she has conscious contact with a higher power and the peace of mind that comes with knowing that things will work out the way they are supposed to.

12. Having had a spiritual awakening as the result of these steps, we tried to carry this message to alcoholics, and to practice these principles in all our affairs. The alcoholic is now transformed from the rigid, angry, controlling person he/she once was to an individual who understands serenity. With a feeling of purpose and usefulness in relationship to the world, the alcoholic becomes altruistic and will now try to help other suffering (or practicing) alcoholics/addicts to achieve sobriety and serenity through their own personal recovery program. In sharing their own experiences, they help other alcoholics stop drinking and/or using drugs while at the same time strengthening their own commitment to sobriety.

The two founders of Alcoholics Anonymous developed the Twelve Steps to help suffering alcoholics achieve a "spiritual awakening" (Alcoholics Anonymous, 1976). Bill Wilson, one of the cofounders of AA, believed that alcoholism was a sickness of the soul that separated man from God. The Twelve Steps began as the key to a spiritual growth experience and served as a guide to recovery for AA, and later many other self-help groups.

From 1970 through 1989, many treatment centers focusing on the treatment of alcoholism were opened. Counselors, who were themselves recovering alcoholics, staffed these centers and chose to use twelve-step principles as the core of their rehabilitation programs because they knew that they worked. Twenty-eight-day style rehabilitation programs typically required clients to finish the first five steps before discharging the clients. The program then referred clients to AA and an AA sponsor to complete the other seven steps. Today's drug and alcohol treatment programs have added other treatment program components but usually a strong emphasis remains on clients attending and integrating into 12-step programs and utilizing the Twelve Steps as the basis for a complete program of recovery in programs that use this model.

In general terms, treatment programs and 12-step groups use the steps and their intended goals as part of the framework for organizing counseling sessions, meetings, and other intervention activities. For example, the first several counseling sessions might focus on the general goal of encouraging the client to accept that he or she has a problem and that old solutions haven't worked—a goal of Step 1. Or the session might include a discussion of how a certain step might be helpful to resolving clients' concerns and day-to-day issues. There are also a number of specific formats designed to help clients learn the twelve-step principles and integrate these principles into their lives. Step study groups run by AA focus on a certain step and discuss its meaning and application to participants' lives. Counselors or sponsors also assign written stepwork as homework assignments that are then discussed and reviewed with clients when they have completed the work. This can take several hours to several days in residential settings to several weeks in an outpatient setting. Some clients need the structure provided by doing the written assignment in session. The client completes each step in order and moves on to the next one when the counselor or sponsor, in consultation with the client, feels that the client's talk and "walk" (behavior) demonstrates some grasp of a given step. The targeted depth of this grasp depends of course on the functional abilities of the client.

Readers familiar with Prochaska and DiClemente's model of change (Prochaska, DiClemente, & Norcross, 1992; discussed in greater detail in Chapter 11 of this volume) might notice a correspondence between the goals of the steps and the various stages of change these researchers had delineated: *contemplation* (Step 1); *preparation* (Steps 1–2); *action* (Steps 3–9); and *maintenance* (Steps 10–12). Readers will also note that the goal is not just abstinence but character transformation through the discipline of working the Twelve Steps.

WORKING A RECOVERY PROGRAM FOR CHEMICAL DEPENDENCE

Chemical dependency counselors often spend time in staff meetings discussing whether or not a client is working a program. There are five key elements to working a recovery program:

1. *Abstinence:* No further ingestion of mind- or mood-altering substances.
2. *Going to meetings:* Regular attendance at 12-step recovery meetings such as AA or NA. Ninety meetings in 90 days is a common suggestion for newly recovering persons.
3. *Working the steps:* Really studying the steps and achieving a psychological, emotional, and spiritual understanding and personal integration of the Twelve Steps. Written stepwork (see Appendix 1 for samples) may be a tool to help familiarize someone with the Twelve Steps.
4. *Sponsorship:* A member of AA or NA with usually 1 or more years of sobriety acts as a guide and mentor to the newly recovering person. Sponsors give ongoing one-on-one feedback to help guide a fellow AA member by sharing their experience, strength, and hope.
5. *Meditation and prayer:* The recovering person's newly developed spirituality is explored and strengthened.

THE MENTAL HEALTH MODEL

Just as with addiction, disease syndrome, learning theory, and psychoanalytic and family therapy paradigms have most influenced the mental health field. And, just as with addiction, a majority of clinicians subscribe to the biopsychosocial model of psychiatric disorders. Although the exact weightings of the factors vary from one disorder to another, this model specifies that psychiatric disorders have *biological, psychological,* and *social* components. These components include both the causes and consequences of each disorder. A corollary of this model is that interventions must address these components in a combined, comprehensive fashion that targets specific components in order to achieve success. For example, schizophrenia appears to be a brain disease with a genetic basis that results in a derangement of both the process and content of thinking as a primary feature. Associated features include oddities in expressed feelings and behavior and impaired interpersonal and role functioning. Highly emotional, demanding interpersonal encounters as well as other stressors can exacerbate the condition. Interventions include medication to improve the process of thinking and the use of structure and skills training to address behavioral deficiencies. Other interventions include working with the family to help them cope with the sick family member. The creation of social support systems helps to maintain and enhance client gains.

As this example illustrates, complex disorders require comprehensive interventions. Mental health providers commonly draw on several sets of strategies and tactics for their interventions, including the following:

1. Mobilizing hope and prompting productive coping through a positive, safe, caring relationship with a therapist or case manager who can give advice and encouragement and facilitate problem solving.
2. Correcting physiological deficiencies through such things as medication, nutritional supplements, and exercise.
3. Building social support systems through such means as attending special issue support groups and mobilizing friendship networks.
4. Addressing existential/spiritual concerns through the discussion of long-term goals, meditation, and encouraging affiliation (or reaffiliation) with various appropriate religious groups.
5. Improving family functioning through such options as education about the disorder, communication skills training, and the negotiation of contracts regarding roles, boundaries, and consequences for specified behaviors.
6. Prompting and reinforcing positive behavior through such tools as reminder cards, behavior checklists, and point systems associated with rewards.
7. Increasing the clients' functional abilities through the teaching of such skills as assertion, stress management, or activities of daily living such as taking the bus or cooking a meal.
8. Encouraging productive thinking patterns through such things as education about the nature of the disorder, using positive self-talk and imagery, or examining faulty assumptions about oneself and others.
9. Increasing client awareness of feelings, thoughts, and behaviors and their interrelationship through such methods as exploring the relationship between family of origin issues and current behavior, commenting on here-and-now behavior in group therapy, and exploring client-created artwork.
10. Decreasing the intensity of unpleasant emotions and other conditioned reactions through reimagining traumatic experiences

and reviewing photo albums to stimulate grief, as well as other abreactive processes.

Selecting and sequencing the appropriate interventions require a careful assessment of the client's current functional level, the manifestation of the specific disorder, and the specific situation of the client. Generally the more acute and/or regressed the client, the earlier in the list mental health professionals start. One way to conceptualize this strategy is to think of it as an *outside-in approach*. At first the provider and the client focus on external and environmental supports and interventions. At this stage the provider and other persons are mainly responsible for treating and supporting the client. Later the provider uses increasingly complex cognitive-behavioral-affective interventions in which the client is a more active agent. As the person improves, higher-order strategies and tactics become more appropriate.

EVALUATION OF SUBSTANCE DEPENDENCE AND DUAL DIAGNOSIS TREATMENT APPROACHES

Numerous evaluations of cognitive-behavioral interventions such as relapse prevention have demonstrated their effectiveness relative to control and some alternative treatments (e.g., Carroll, 1996; Miller et al., 1995).

Historically there has been relatively little empirical evidence for the efficacy of 12-step program approaches. This unfortunate shortcoming has recently been remedied, however.

Wells, Peterson, Gainey, Hawkins, and Catalano (1994) compared 12-step and relapse prevention psychotherapy groups for cocaine-dependent outpatients. Both groups showed reductions in chemical use, with no appreciable differences at posttreatment on cocaine or marijuana use.

Project Match (Project Match Research Group, 1997) compared cognitive-behavioral coping skills, motivational enhancement, and 12-step facilitation treatments in large samples of inpatient and outpatient alcohol-dependent clients recruited nationwide. The study used well-written treatment manuals and certified therapists in all three approaches to ensure fidelity to the treatment approaches. The study also employed intensive efforts to retain the clients in treatment, such as reminder letters and follow-up phone calls for missed appointments. Under these ideal conditions, rates of abstinence in general were greater than 80% at 1-year follow-up, with little significant difference among types of treatments. A prime aim of the project was to ascertain whether clients with certain characteristics did better with one particular type of treatment or another. Of the many characteristics studied, only psychiatric severity demonstrated a robust interaction effect with type of treatment. Clients low in psychiatric severity had more abstinent days in 12-step facilitation treatment than with cognitive-behavioral therapy. Neither treatment was superior for clients with higher levels of psychiatric severity. Clients who were higher in "meaning seeking" at intake (that is, they complained of perceiving little meaning in life and aspired to experience greater meaning) were somewhat more responsive to 12-step facilitation than to other treatments. Certain client characteristics did predict treatment outcomes in a very modest way. Males and those with higher psychiatric severity had fewer abstinent days. Once a subject began drinking, being male, having a high original involvement with alcohol and high social support for drinking, and psychiatric severity predicted a higher number of drinks per drinking day. Greater sociopathy was associated with worse outcomes early in follow-up but not later. A later analysis of the same data showed that clients who had social support networks that promoted drinking did better if they went to AA and that 12-step facilitation did a better job of getting these clients to attend AA at 3-year follow-up (Longabaugh, Wirtz, Zweben, & Stout, 1998). Readers should note that none of the treatments offered any education directly about the disease of addiction (as is commonly done in treatment programs nowadays) and that, while participants were encouraged to attend outside 12-step meetings, this was not a requirement.

Another large-scale evaluation of treatment outcomes for inpatient treatment programs in the U.S. Department of Veterans Affairs Medical Centers compared 12-step and cognitive-behavioral treatments for substance abuse (Ouimettte, Finney, & Moos, 1997). While 12-step patients were more likely to be abstinent at 1-year follow-up, generally 12-step, cognitive-behavioral, and combined 12-step/cognitive-behavioral programs were equally effective in reducing substance use and improving most other areas of functioning. Patients with only substance abuse diagnoses, those with concomitant psychiatric diagnoses, and those who were involuntarily mandated to receive treatment showed equivalent outcomes. It should be noted that only 25% of patients were in complete remission at follow-up, and high levels of anxiety, depression, and unemployment were common. Interestingly, a later analysis of the same data showed that 12-step treatments did the same or better than cognitive-behavioral treatments in changing the input variables thought to be associated with change in the cognitive-behavioral framework (Finney, Noyes, Coutts, & Moos, 1998).

McKay et al. (1997) compared standard group counseling with a 12-step focus against individualized relapse prevention featuring aftercare for cocaine-dependent clients completing a standard intensive outpatient program. Rates of complete abstinence during the 6 month study period were higher for the standard group counseling. Relapse prevention reduced the extent of use of those who used during the first 3 months, with no difference between treatments after that. Lifetime diagnoses of alcohol dependence, major depression, and any anxiety disorder predicted less cocaine use (similar to the results of other studies of cocaine abusers cited by McKay et al.), and antisocial personality disorder had no relationship to outcome.

As is evident from many of the studies cited above, the past decade has seen increasing appreciation of the role of psychiatric comorbidity with substance use disorders. However, most of these studies, while using comorbid psychiatric diagnoses as a predictor of treatment outcome, did not measure or systematically vary the psychiatric services received (if any) by the addicted clients with coexisting psychiatric disorders. What about studies directly concerned with clients with dual disorders?

Two early uncontrolled studies indicated decreased days of hospitalization for program members receiving treatment for both disorders (Hellerstein & Meehan, 1987; Kofoed, Kania, Walsh, & Atkinson, 1986).

In one of the first controlled studies, Woody, O'Brien, McLellan, and Evans (1982) demonstrated that antidepressant medications were helpful for methadone-maintained clients with persistent symptoms of major depression. Woody, McLellan, and Luborsky (1984) later demonstrated that adding psychotherapy to standard alcohol and drug counseling, while having no appreciable impact on chemically dependent persons with low psychiatric severity, substantially improved the results of treatment for patients with moderate and, most especially, those with high psychiatric severity scores.

McLellan et al. (1994) did a large-scale correlational study of opiate-, alcohol-, and cocaine-dependent male and female adults treated in inpatient and outpatient settings in 22 publicly and privately funded programs. Outcomes were predicted by similar factors regardless of drug problem or setting. Greater substance use at follow-up was predicted only by the greater severity of substance use at admission, not by the number of services received during treatment, with the authors suggesting a possible ceiling effect (observable whenever effects have reached their highest limit) to account for these somewhat surprising results. More serious employment, family, and, especially, psychiatric problems at admission predicted more severe problems after treatment, with the effect stronger for social adjustment outcomes than substance use outcomes. The more psychiatric, family, employment, and medical services provided during treatment (but not substance abuse services), the better the social adjustment. There was little relationship between these services and substance use outcomes.

Swindle, Phibbs, Paradise, Recine, & Moos (1995) did a national study of Veterans Administration Medical Center dually diagnosed inpatients to determine what factors facilitated decreased readmissions, specifically comparing dual diagnosis units with dual diagnosis groups in alcohol and drug treatment units. Findings indicated that dual diagnosis treatment that had an integrated, primary disease–recovery focus and used "tolerant persuasion" to deal with relapses were more successful. Programs that had staff-led rather than peer-oriented groups and that provided continuity of staff in aftercare also had better outcomes.

Jerrell and Ridgely (1995) used a quasi-experimental design and compared 12-step recovery, behavioral skills training, and intensive case management interventions for clients with severe mental illness and substance use disorders over a 24-month period. The study found modest positive changes for many of the psychosocial outcomes, although the rates of change in alcohol and drug use were small to none. The study found that behavioral skills were a more effective treatment than case management interventions and that both were more effective than 12-step intervention in reducing psychiatric and chemical use symptoms and improving social functioning. The 12-step recovery intervention included transitional AA meeting groups at the mental health center, taking clients to AA meetings and attempting to facilitate the development of a sponsor, and generally providing supportive counseling in the 12-step process. The behavioral skills training taught clients self-management skills, including drug and alcohol relapse prevention skills. The intensive case management approach involved intensive assistance with all life areas as well as some educational sessions on alcohol and drug effects and ways of preventing a relapse. The authors note difficulties in consistently implementing the interventions.

Drake, Mueser, Clark, and Wallach (1996) reviewed studies of dual diagnosis treatment with clients suffering severe mental illness. Their original findings indicated some pessimism. For example, the National Institute of Mental Health funded 13 dual diagnosis demonstration projects between 1987 and 1990, with most of the studies having only a 1-year follow-up and no control groups. A review of these studies (Mercer-McFadden & Drake, 1995, as quoted in Drake, Mueser, Clark, & Wallach, 1996) reached these conclusions: (1) engagement rates were high (75–85%); (2) utilization rates of inpatient and institutional services decreased; (3) there was minimal or no reduction in substance abuse; (4) dually diagnosed clients were not motivated to participate in the abstinence-based treatment programs offered. However, Drake et al. also indicated that the preliminary findings from uncontrolled studies of treatment programs that provided integrated (as opposed to parallel treatments) and that had longer follow-up periods did demonstrate that many clients could attain some degree of abstinence and that there are also dramatic reductions in hospitalization and significant improvements in functioning.

Finally, Cox et al. (1998) in a study of homeless alcoholics (with high rates of dual diagnosis) demonstrated that intensive case management resulted in improved financial and residential stability and reduced alcohol use.

BEST-PRACTICE INTERVENTIONS

What approaches are available to the counselor or case manager seeking to select effective interventions for the client with dual disorders? There is no magic, 100% effective approach, but treatment can make a difference. Furthermore, the past decade of research supports the wisdom of undertaking to implement the following specific recommendations: (1) integrating substance dependence and mental health interventions in one setting and program; (2) providing an array of both substance abuse and mental health treatment services to address the multiplicity of problems presented by clients with dual disorders (and not just referring to a 12-step program); (3) providing for continuity of care and case management; (4) promoting the notion of recovery to both staff and clients as an ongoing process that will take time in demonstrating change; (5) having tolerant policies toward use and relapse that walk the line between enabling and rigidity; (6)utilizing interventions drawn from either 12-step or cognitive-behavioral interventions but making sure to include or provide abstinence as the goal, education about the disease model, and sober support at follow-up.

Next we will delineate a detailed integrated model for treating dually diagnosed clients.

CHAPTER 3

An Integrated Model of Dual Recovery

Religion is for those who fear going to hell;
spirituality is for those who have already been there.
—ANONYMOUS

In this chapter we detail our own integrated model for working with clients with dual disorders, and we argue for its utility. We discuss some solutions to problems associated with integrating mental health and with chemical dependency treatment in general and in regard to treatment from within a 12-step recovery model in particular. We also discuss organizational issues that arise in implementing dual diagnosis programs and suggest possible solutions for dealing with these barriers. Finally, we provide a brief discourse on managed health care and dual diagnosis treatment.

A RECOVERY-BASED APPROACH FOR TREATING CLIENTS WITH DUAL DISORDERS

Dually diagnosed clients suffer from coexisting independent disorders that require simultaneous integrated intervention in order to achieve the best outcomes. Our general strategy for doing this is to blend recovery model notions with mental health ones.

We first believe that the recovery model and the mental health model have many similarities that can serve to unite chemical dependency and mental health professionals and that also can keep things simple for clients and their families. Table 1 contains more detailed comparisons between various aspects of the recovery and the mental health models.

TABLE 1. Selected Comparisons of the Recovery and the Mental Health Models

Recovery model	Mental health model
Disease process	Syndrome concept
Biopsychosocial and spiritual factors	Biopsychosocial factors
	Some attention to philosophical issues
Chronic condition	Chronic condition of most major disorders
Relapse issues	Relapse issues
Genetic/physiological component	Genetic/physiological component in most disorders
Chemical use primary	Psychiatric disorder primary
Out of control	Ineffective coping
Denial	Poor insight
Despair	Demoralization
Family issues	Family issues
Social stigma	Social stigma
Abstinence early goal	Stability early goal
Recovery long-term goal	Rehabilitation long-term goal
Powerlessness	Empowerment
No use of mood-altering chemicals	Psychotropic medications used
Education about illness	Education about illness
Halfway houses, ALANO clubs	Group homes, day treatment
Sponsors	Case manager or therapist
AA, Al-Anon, self-help groups	Support groups
Concrete action	Behavior change
Self-examination and acceptance	Awareness and insight
Label self as alcoholic/addict	See self as whole person with a disorder
Practice of communication and social skills	Practice of communication and social skills
Slogans, stories, affirmations	Positive self-talk, imagery
Stepwork	Psychotherapy
Use of spiritual concepts	Use of existential, transpersonal, some spiritual concepts
Family therapy	Family therapy
Group and individual work	Group and individual work
Continuum of care	Continuum of care
Nutrition, exercise, growth as value	Wellness concepts

Close inspection of this table reveals that many of the two models' concepts are exactly the same or (after taking into account differences in language and emphasis) very similar. For example, both models are grounded in a biopsychosocial framework. Both look at genetic bases and disease processes, seek to modify attitudes and defenses, and emphasize the importance of social support and family involvement. Both models use many psychotherapy techniques. The AA slogan of "one day at a time" is a wonderful cognitive restructuring intervention, for example. The mental health notion of attitudes following behavior is highly compatible with the recovery notion of "fake it 'til you make it." Correcting chemical imbalances resulting from excessive alcohol use with nutritional supplements is conceptually similar to correcting such imbalances with lithium carbonate in bipolar disorders.

The two approaches can share the same general goal of recovery and can use an outside-in, first-things-first, treatment strategy. The priority for early stages of recovery from chemical dependency is simply maintaining abstinence, and typically the interventions rely on frequent AA meetings, calling sponsors, and looking at "stinkin' thinkin,'" that is, attitudes signaling relapse. Later chemical dependency work relies on stepwork to achieve positive aspects of health through addressing issues such as guilt, fear, and resentment. Similarly, the priority in the early stages of recovery from psychiatric disorders is simply maintaining stability, and typically interventions rely on case management, a structured lifestyle, and acceptance of the need to manage the disorder. Later mental health work relies on skills training and psychotherapy to achieve positive functioning through addressing issues such as grief at having an illness, establishing intimacy, and operating as a prosocial member of society. We quite easily and comfortably say that *the goal of treatment for our dually diagnosed clients is dual recovery*, that is, recovery from both disorders.

The two approaches can also complement each other. Education in the disease concept, stepwork, and involvement in AA require the ability to process information, to tolerate painful emotions, and to relate effectively to others. Knowledge of the neuropsychological impairment associated with different psychiatric disorders, ways to work with different psychological defenses, and behavioral skill training techniques to prompt prorecovery behavior can be invaluable in doing chemical dependency work with dually diagnosed clients. Those suffering from schizophrenia, for example, are more impaired in auditory–verbal information processing and benefit more from visual–motor means of presenting information. Borderlines, typically survivors of traumatic childhood abuse, benefit from Step 4 work (making "a

searching and fearless moral inventory") that focuses on current resentments and avoids dredging up traumatic childhood memories.
Providing anxiety-management skills to the client with an anxiety disorder can help ensure that the client will get out of the house and to
AA meetings.

Similarly, the recovery model can help fine-tune mental health approaches to certain issues. Concern with preventing relapse is relevant
not only to chemical use problems but also to such problems as noncompliance with medications and recurrent major depressions or episodic
cutting. The progressive structure and achievements of stepwork and the
encouragement of positive action often give depressed persons a behavioral lift that they desperately need. Using Step 1 notions of powerlessness
and unmanageability can help persons with a bipolar disorder accept the
need for treatment through examining failed attempts at willpower-based
self-control and the negative impact of unmanaged bipolar disorder on
their lives.

We continue to use a 12-step recovery framework for that and other
reasons as the overall thematic backdrop to our treatment approach.
We feel that abstinence must be the goal of treatment for clients with
dual disorders. Twelve-step-based approaches have abstinence as the
goal of treatment and appear to promote this goal more effectively than
other types of interventions. The disease concept provides a nonjudgmental, easy-to-understand rationale for the need to abstain. The
concept also helps clients with dual diagnoses reframe their sense of
self from being bad to being sick and reinforces education about their
second disease or syndrome, the psychiatric disorder. Moreover, research indicates that long-term success at recovery is not especially associated with time-limited treatment but rather with increased positive
events related to abstinence and decreased negative events in general
during early recovery (Tucker, Vuchinich, & Pukish, 1995). Affiliation
with Alcoholics Anonymous can serve as a potent relapse preventer by
enhancing self-efficacy and motivation and increasing efforts at coping over a long period of time (Morgenstern et al., 1997). Treatment
within the recovery model can assist clients in learning the culture of
AA and making use of this free, widely available, and easily accessible
ongoing support. The AA notion of "recovering, not recovered" reinforces the need for long-term attention to maintaining any gains made
and for contingency plans for managing relapse. Working the Twelve
Steps of Alcoholics Anonymous provides a "philosophy of living" that
fosters attitudes and skills that promote not just coping but personal
growth as well. Finally, 12-step programs address the existential and
spiritual issues that persons with dual disorders face.

COGNITIVE-BEHAVIORAL APPROACHES

While we use the 12-step recovery model as the foundation of our approach, we also rely on cognitive-behavioral approaches as well (e.g., Carroll, 1996; Kadden et al., 1994; Monti, Abrams, Kadden, & Cooney, 1989). We find that they blend smoothly and easily into our overall dual recovery framework; moreover, they have strong empirical support. Consequently, we will spend some time discussing these in more detail.

Cognitive-behavioral approaches focus on thinking and behavior as the targets for change. The first strategy typically employed is to help the client identify high-risk situations for drinking or using by employing an ABC model. *A* stands for antecedents or cues and triggers for behavior. These cues can be external or they can be internal (such as cravings). *B* is for behavior and is defined broadly to include thoughts, feelings, physiological reactions, and overt behavior. *C* is for consequences, or the rewarding or punishing effects of the behavior. Counselors work with clients to identify the ABCs of their drinking or using behavior through questions, roleplays, or the review of journals kept by clients. The second strategy is to help the client plan and practice alternatives. It is crucial to have clients identify what they are going to think and do *instead* of drinking and using. Too many clients have a "Don't use" program. This "negative" plan is not by itself likely to be a firm basis for sustained recovery—for a variety of reasons. One reason is the "Don't think of pink elephants" phenomenon. The more one tries *not* to think a particular thought, the more likely one is to think it! And so it goes with "Don't drink, don't drink, don't drink." Another reason is that the *motivation* is purely negative. While holding on to the negative consequences of using is important, so is focusing on the positive consequences of recovery.

A number of tactics fall under the rubric of "alternatives." One set of tactics involves avoiding high-risk situations. Another set of tactics is to challenge faulty beliefs about substance use, such as the belief that it's the only way to have fun or that the substance is relaxing (as opposed to merely relieving withdrawal symptoms). A third set of tactics is to help clients learn new skills to manage feelings (such as relaxation skills) or to function more effectively (such as through assertiveness) or to say no to offers of chemicals (refusal skills). A final set of tactics is to change the consequences for the behavior, such as losing a job for continued use or helping clients obtain monetary rewards for staying clean. Always the emphasis is on utilization of new information and skills through roleplaying, imagery exercises (wherein one plays a "movie" of the new skill in imagination), and homework assignments.

One specific example of a behavioral intervention that we use quite extensively is the fail-safe card. Using index cards, we have clients write out possible triggers for symptomatic behavior on one side and three or four simple prorecovery responses on the other. These latter might include checking with the psychiatrist about medication or calling a sponsor. We then encourage clients to carry these cards around in their wallets as a kind of "therapist in a pocket," a phrase used by one of our clients.

RELAPSE PREVENTION

Relapse is very common among dually diagnosed clients and needs to be a focus in treatment, preferably sooner rather than later. For example, one study of remission of substance use disorders among psychiatric inpatients found that, while 26% had apparently achieved remission from a previous substance use disorder, 46% of patients at admission had a substance use disorder and many continued to relapse through 1-year follow-up, (Dixon, McNary, & Lehman, 1998). The best predictor of relapse for addictive behaviors and a number of psychiatric disorders is the experience of negative emotional states and negative life events (Doering, Muller, Kopcke, Peitzcker, & Gaebael, 1998; Johnson & Miller, 1997; Kessler, 1997; Brennan & Moos, 1990). Low availability of social support and poor quality of social support are also associated with relapse for both chemical dependency and psychiatric disorders (Erickson, Beiser, & Iacono, 1998; O'Farrell, Hooley, Fals-Stewart, & Cutter, 1998; Fenton, Blyler, & Heinssen, 1997; Tucker et al., 1995; Brennan & Moos, 1990).

Some research evidence indicates that there may be a tendency wherein relapse prevention strategies end up *lowering* the absolute rates of abstinence (McKay et al., 1997; Ouimette et al., 1997; Carroll, 1996). Evidence for a variety of interventions in reducing relapse of psychiatric disorders such as major depressive, bipolar, and schizophrenic disorders is similarly mixed and confusing (e.g., Gortner, Gollan, Dobson, & Jacobson, 1998; Fenton et al., 1997; Parikh et al., 1997). Perhaps this is because focusing on relapse may implicitly give permission for substance use to occur. Discussions of relapse have the capacity to backfire, since, for example, persons with a major depression might even see more reason to feel hopeless and suggestible trauma survivors might simply decide to take the counselor up on the implied suggestion and introspect unduly and unwisely.

Given the high probability of dual relapses among clients, however, addressing this crucial subject of relapse prevention planning directly—using both cognitive-behavioral techniques and the tactics of 12-step programs—is beneficial. As with blending substance abuse and mental health treatment in general, there is no inherent or unresolvable conflict between these two approaches. Twelve-step recovery approaches give out special coins or tokens for 30 days of sobriety as a "reward through recognition" while cognitive-behavioral approaches advise one to develop a sober support system, or network of supportive friends. We use these kinds of strategies while emphasizing the disease and need-for-abstinence messages with our dually diagnosed clients.

Blending addict recovery and mental health approaches does raise several controversial issues, however—some relating to the chemical dependency field in general and others to the dual diagnosis field in particular. Below we discuss these controversies and offer resolutions that we think help to make the marriage work.

CONTROVERSIES

Primary versus Secondary

The first controversial issue is the *primary–secondary* one, a distinction used in several ways. As noted earlier, the traditional mental health view of chemical abuse and dependency holds that these problems are symptoms of an underlying psychiatric disorder. Although it acknowledges the need to manage withdrawal symptoms and other serious concomitants of the chemical use, this view holds that the psychiatric disorder is the primary target for treatment. People who meet the criteria for substance abuse but not dependency (with loss of control, withdrawal) are especially likely to be treated within this framework. Similarly, the traditional chemical dependency view holds that the chemical involvement is the root of the individual's problems and that achieving abstinence and working a recovery program are all that the person needs to do. Although it acknowledges the need to manage severe symptoms such as psychosis or self-harm with additional measures, this view holds that the client's chemical use must be the main focus of treatment. People who demonstrate only subtle signs of depression and anxiety are especially likely to be treated within this framework.

Another way that professionals deal with the primary–secondary distinction is to prioritize the sequence of treatment. Although the psychiatric disorder or the chemical use is accepted as an independent problem, the more emergent problem requires primary attention. Only after a significant period of psychiatric stability (or, alternatively, abstinence) does the chemical use or dependency (or psychiatric disorder) merit treatment. Treatment in such cases as these is more sequential than simultaneous.

We again stress the notion of *coexisting disorders* and the need for *simultaneous treatment*. We believe that some people who have problematic chemical involvements may also have an independent psychiatric disorder, and vice versa. As we have already seen, a psychiatric disorder confers no immunity for chemical abuse and dependency and, in fact, appears to increase the risk of developing these difficulties. The converse also appears to be true. In addition, the synergistic effect of both sets of problems makes treating first one set of problems and attaining abstinence or psychiatric stability difficult. The provider must therefore usually manage and treat both problems simultaneously.

A corollary to this stance is the crucial importance of a comprehensive assessment of all clients to identify those with dual disorders. Approximately half of all psychiatric clients have symptoms related to substance use, and about half of all substance abusers have psychiatric symptoms (Osher, 1996). Since problematic chemical involvements can produce difficulties that mimic a host of psychiatric disorders, the challenge for the provider is often to establish the existence of the psychiatric disorder. For this purpose of differential diagnosis, a modified primary–secondary distinction may be useful (Schuckit, 1986). Nonetheless, when providers identify dual disorders, they must give equal weight to the chemical use and the psychiatric disorders. In Chapter 5, we discuss these issues in more detail.

Abuse versus Dependence

The distinctions between *substance abuse versus substance dependence* can be controversial. Persons who are dependent, by definition, cannot control their use of the substance in question. Abstinence must then be the goal. On the other hand, persons who "abuse" chemicals can presumably learn to moderate their use or use them in a way that minimizes negative consequences.

We believe that the distinction is not a useful one for dually diagnosed clients. As we argue further in the next section, abstinence must be the goal for these persons.

Abstinence versus Controlled Use

One controversial difference in the chemical dependency treatment field involves the goal of intervention. Should professionals and programs emphasize *total abstinence* from all mood-altering chemicals, or should *controlled use* be the goal of interventions? In the literature on controlled use these discussions typically focus on alcohol use. Few professionals would advocate the controlled use of heroin or crack, although we have occasionally encountered a counselor or case manager who feels that controlled use of marijuana is relatively benign. Professionals arguing for controlled use have typically made a distinction between problem users and true alcoholics and addicts, cite studies showing controlled use by formerly alcoholic or addicted persons, or generally feel that it is better to attempt this goal with clients unwilling to accept abstinence than to have troubled clients receive no help at all (Rosenberg, 1993).

We believe that *abstinence* (from addictive drugs) must be the goal of treatment for clients with dual disorders, while also acknowledging that this may take some time. Even for singly diagnosed alcoholics (never mind dually diagnosed clients who are substance dependent), the available research and the bulk of professional opinion indicate that controlled drinking is impossible and dangerous for substance-dependent alcoholics (e.g., Wallace, 1996). Indeed, loss of control is a cardinal feature of substance dependence. We advocate abstinence even for those dually diagnosed clients who are merely "abusing" chemicals ("merely" only in the sense that they have *some* choice in the matter). Even assuming one can even make a clear distinction between problem users versus addicts in this population, clients with a psychiatric disorder are at increased risk of developing a substance use disorder and of having ongoing problems with chemicals even with treatment. Individuals already suffering from disordered brain chemistry due to a psychiatric disorder do not need to contribute to the problem by ingesting intoxicating substances. Drinking on top of medication is not advised. We believe that any use of psychoactive chemicals by someone with a psychiatric disorder is at least misuse and routinely ask for an abstinence agreement even from our psychiatric-diagnosis-only clients. Their response to the request and their compliance with their agreement are often quite revealing. Early counseling contacts can establish that a dialogue about substance use will certainly be part of the treatment agenda.

Readiness for Treatment
and Confrontation versus Enabling

Another controversial issue involves *readiness for treatment*. Some professionals refuse to accept clients who appear to lack internal motivation and the willingness or "the desire to stop drinking." Perhaps the AA belief that alcoholics must hit bottom and surrender before they are willing to change and certainly frustrating experiences with clients in denial have both contributed to this attitude. Recent research and conceptual developments have somewhat softened many providers' stance on this issue, however. For example, studies have shown no difference in outcome for mandated versus voluntary adult clients treated in alcohol and drug programs (Ouimette et al., 1997; Watson, Brown, Tilleskjor, Jacobs, & Purcel, 1988). The development of intervention strategies (Liepman, 1993), motivational interviewing (Miller & Rollnick, 1991), and the stages-of-change model (Prochaska et al., 1992) has increased the sophistication of professionals in understanding and intervening with individuals who have less than ideal motivation for chemical dependency treatment. Nonetheless, the issue remains a controversial one. Some professionals still insist on clients "doing it my way, right now" and otherwise not admitting these clients to treatment or discharging them immediately. Our experience has also been that some managed health care reviewers are highly reluctant to pay for contemplation-stage counseling and sometimes issue an ultimatum that the client "go to a meeting this week" or else they will stop paying for treatment.

The *role of confrontation* in treatment for substance abuse disorders is an issue related to the readiness-for-treatment one. Probably most strongly associated in people's minds with the 1970s Synanon program for heroin addicts, the use of "tough love" with alcoholics and addicts and harsh confrontation of their behavior in order to break through denial is strongly advocated by some professionals. Critics have seen the casualties of these interventions and have rightly questioned both the ethics and efficacy of "in your face" as a therapeutic tool, particularly with clients with dual disorders. Some recent research has even demonstrated that the confrontation can result in increased use in alcohol-dependent clients (Miller, Benefield, & Tonigan, 1993). Such critics sometimes fail to understand that Synanon-style confrontations normally take place in the context of a therapeutic community and with clients with strong antisocial defenses. On the other hand, a neutral or nondirective style with a practicing alcoholic or addict may also prove problematic. Such clients are likely to be adept at redefining the problem or otherwise rationalizing and justifying their activities. The treatment goes nowhere and the clients' clinical status continues to deteriorate. The *confrontation versus enabling* issue remains divisive.

We believe in *flexible but direct challenges* to the denial system of clients with dual disorders. Ignoring clients' substance use or equivocating in treatment is not helpful. Nor is simply pounding away at persons suffering from severe depression or psychotic symptoms. We do believe that being honest and straightforward in our concerns is respectful not only of our need to proceed responsibly and professionally but also of our clients' need and right to be treated as the persons ultimately responsible for their own health and life. We also believe that professionals can time and titrate the intensity of their interventions according to clients' clinical status and overall situation. Lack of insight and motivation is a clinical issue, and appropriate interventions are warranted. We might either explicitly negotiate three sessions to further explore the situation further with a client willing to give a time-limited no-use contract or recommend more intensive residential treatment for someone who continues to "not get it." Chapter 11 explores the issue of motivation in more detail.

Facilitator versus Mentor

We have sometimes witnessed disagreement around another aspect of therapist style, namely, whether the therapist is to be a *specialist facilitator or a personal mentor* to clients. For clinicians trained in certain mental health therapy approaches, the ideal therapist is to be a blank screen for clients to project their issues onto, providing a forum for the therapist to identify and comment on the clients' issues. Or the ideal therapist is completely and totally congruent and at one with clients and always lets clients go where they want to go in order to facilitate self-exploration. In contrast, the recovery approach (perhaps because so many of its early champions were recovering themselves) has modeled a therapy style based on the AA role of sponsor. The ideal therapist then is like the ideal sponsor: recovering, self-disclosing, available as needed, and the teacher/master to the client/pupil of how to do recovery in general and how to work the Twelve Steps in particular.

We advocate for an *active but professional style* with clients. We believe that effective treatment with dually diagnosed clients requires vigorous engagement with clients and energetic implementation of a treatment plan. Addiction and even many mental health disorders are potentially fatal and certainly disruptive and damaging. Effective interventions are available. Passively waiting for something to happen is inappropriate treatment. On the other hand, we are treatment providers, not sponsors. While in-depth knowledge of recovery concepts is necessary, being an alcoholic or addict in recovery is not—nor is personal experience a qualification for providing treatment. Personal and program boundaries are important. A limited amount of self-disclosure, with clients who are not psychotic or who do not have acting-out personality disorders and when not a reflection of the therapist's own needs, can be useful at decreasing shame and providing hope. Recovering counselors are going to have to work out such issues as how they will respond, for example, when clients go to the same AA meetings that they attend. There need to be decisions about such matters as the availability of after-hours on-call support and the like.

Psychotropic Medications

The use of *psychotropic medications* is another point of potential controversy. In the past some medical professionals have created iatrogenic addictions with such medications as the benzodiazepines or have inadvertently substituted such medications for alcohol. Some members of the 12-step community recall being detoxed with benzodiazepines and think that all psychotropic medications are of this nature. They might then advise clients with dual disorders that "a drug is a drug" and that they discontinue the prescribed medication. Professionals or concerned laypeople wonder about mixed messages, with one message being "Do life drug-free" and the other being "Take this drug."

We absolutely refuse to recommend or condone the use of addictive medications after detoxification. The dangers of cross-addiction and the importance of a chemical-free lifestyle for dually diagnosed clients make this a crucial issue. But we are quite comfortable *using appropriate psychotropic medications* after a comprehensive evaluation indicates that the client requires this for his/her psychiatric disorder and/or after non-pharmacologic interventions have not worked. Medication helps the seriously mentally ill client become available for engaging in a recovery program. In fact, we believe that failure to prescribe medications when indicated for a psychiatric disorder constitutes malpractice. The opioids, stimulants, benzodiazepines, barbiturates, and other sedative-hypnotics are potentially addictive; with these exceptions, the other standard psychotropic medications are not especially addictive. In fact, the issue is usually convincing clients to take or to stay on these medications! There is often a substantial time lag between taking these medications and any relief, and many of these medications have annoying and troubling side effects. For example, many clients experience loss of sexual interest and significant weight gain on some of the antidepressants. Most of the psychotropics are just not a lot of fun. We do make sure that the client understands and works through the difference between appropriate medication and medications and substances with abuse potential. With less regressed clients, we encourage them to be honest with their own physicians about their problems with addiction. We work with physicians to avoid p. r. n. (taken as needed) medication instructions to minimize the connection between immediate distress and taking a pill. We work with clients to develop alternative skills for relief. We also help clients to learn to handle any challenges to their medication use by a member of a 12-step support group.

Twelve-Step Programs Are Inappropriate for Dually Diagnosed Clients

The involvement of dually diagnosed clients in AA or NA and with a sponsor is sometimes a source of controversy. Developed originally for single diagnosis alcoholics, *12-step programs might be inappropriate for clients with dual disorders*, say critics. Concerns revolve around the ability of some dually diagnosed clients (e. g., the individual with paranoid symptoms) to tolerate meetings. Other concerns include instances where an AA member has challenged the client's use of psychotropic medication or has accused the client of not working the program when the client discusses his/her psychiatric symptoms. Survivors of childhood abuse often experience a severe crisis when prematurely attempting a Step 4 (the "fearless moral moral inventory"), and Step 2 (belief in "a power greater than ourselves") can inappropriately reinforce religious delusions. One must constantly remember that, helpful as they may be, 12-step programs are not treatment or a substitute for treatment.

We strongly urge our dually diagnosed clients *to attend self-help recovery groups*. These groups offer readily available, free social support that can help dually diagnosed clients to maintain not only abstinence but also psychiatric stability. Moreover, these groups also help these individuals with such problems as social isolation, poor social skills, low rates of productive behavior, and distorted patterns of thinking that are associated with their disorders. Some AA and NA groups and sponsors are remarkably tolerant and accepting of the special issues and needs of the dually diagnosed. In the larger metropolitan areas there are also now Dual Recovery and Double Trouble 12-step groups. Others have developed special self-help groups that are a blend of 12-step and group therapy that serve as a substitute or transition group for dually diagnosed persons (e.g., Hasting-Vertino, 1996). Although we find less need to do this now than we did 10 years ago, we do work with dually diagnosed individuals to prepare them for possible challenges to their mental health treatment. We also work with clients to develop the attitudes and skills necessary to first tolerate and then adapt to the meeting process. We explain that AA and NA have no official position on the use of medications and that a gentle response of "work your own program" is often all that is needed to silence amateur clinicians. AA also has a pamphlet available titled "On medications" that reinforces our efforts in this area. We will also hold mock meetings, go on trial runs for meetings, meet with sponsors, and coach our clients and their spouses to increase comfort levels. We help clients locate supportive meetings and/or sponsors or start such meetings. Finally, we employ modified stepwork with our dually diagnosed clients that takes into account the assets, liabilities, and processes that are part of their particular psychiatric disorder. As Chapters 5 and 6 explain in more detail, our experience is that dually diagnosed clients not only can do, and benefit from, stepwork for their chemical use issues but also for their psychiatric disorders as well.

Labeling

The recovery model also strongly encourages clients to *accept the label of alcoholic or addict.* Some professionals see the insistence that dually diagnosed clients label themselves as alcoholics or addicts as detrimental to clients' self-esteem. We would argue that the acceptance of the label and acknowledgment of this to self and others is therapeutic. We would also argue, incidentally, that this is valid for the psychiatric disorder as well. "My name is *X* and I am an alcoholic and schizophrenic" is a statement in which *the label can be liberating.* Clients' acceptance of their difficulties is a prerequisite for management of their disorder. Public acknowledgment of the situation also combats the denial of others and the stigma associated with these disorders. Clients who see themselves as *only* their label need help with this in sessions. A public that reduces clients *only* to their label needs education.

Powerlessness versus Empowerment

Many professionals have difficulty with the recovery concept of *powerlessness versus the empowerment concept* that much of their training has emphasized. Don't we minimize strengths and assets and undercut clients' sense of self-efficacy if we ask them to admit powerlessness and to surrender? As we discussed earlier in this chapter in the review of Step 1 and its meaning, powerlessness and empowerment are not necessarily conflicting concepts. In working with dually diagnosed clients, our goal is to *empower them through surrender* by taking responsibility for their own thinking, emotions, and behavior. Powerlessness is a paradox in our view. By letting go of old, unsuccessful ways of controlling, under controlling, and over controlling chemical use (and in some cases their psychiatric disorders), individuals can learn to relax, gain peace of mind, and begin to manage their disorders and live in a more productive fashion.

Spirituality

Spirituality is a final controversial issue. "Let go and let God" is an AA slogan often heard in meetings, and meetings conclude with the Lord's Prayer. Phrases such as "power greater than ourselves" and "God, as we

understood Him" raise fears about an attempt to convert the dually diagnosed client to a particular religion or view of God. Members of AA and
NA are very clear that this Higher Power is an individual choice and can
be anyone or anything that could be a positive force in the individual's
life. The concept is simply an attempt to assist the suffering alcoholic or
addict in understanding that (1) he/she is not alone; (2) there is help;
(3) things will improve; and (4) willpower alone will not stop the addictive
behavior. These are valuable lessons for dealing with many psychiatric
disorders, as well. Individuals with a thought disorder pose particular
challenges when using Higher Power concepts. It is not uncommon for
these individuals to have religious delusions where, for example, they
believe that they alone hear the voice of God. We discourage discussions
of a Higher Power with someone with religious delusions, of course taking into account individual and cultural values when trying to determine
whether the person's notions are delusional. We employ a practical approach in which we keep discussions concrete and focus on *having clients
develop a sense of faith by looking at how things are better today than yesterday
and how something or someone else can help.* The specialized stepwork in
appendix 1 illustrates our approach to these issues.

PROGRAMMATIC INTEGRATION OF TREATMENT

The overall success of a dual diagnosis program depends heavily on effective organizational integration of treatment. Whether the program is
being instituted in an inpatient unit or in an outpatient program, a clear
structure and consistent philosophy must emanate from the administrative level. In the early stages of developing a dual diagnosis program,
when either converting a traditional chemical dependency program to
dual diagnosis or implementing a dual diagnosis treatment in a psychiatric unit or in a mental health setting, it is essential to develop a clear
philosophy and mission statement around which the program staff can
organize.

Implementing the coexisting-disorders-requiring-simultaneous-
treatment model requires a philosophy statement that is consistent with
this theme. Administrative personnel need to speak, write, and demonstrate that this is the mission of their program. It is useful to establish a
strong message at the start so that those members of the treatment team
who aren't comfortable with that philosophy can either become more
comfortable or choose another agency or facility to work in where there
is a better philosophical and theoretical match.

An administrator or program director who gives an unclear or wishy-
washy message will establish a climate for much professional and personal

conflict among staff members. This is not to suggest that an overly controlling stance needs to be taken by the individual in charge. Rather, the boss needs to give a consistent message about the mission of the program and to be a strong supporter of staff members trying to carry out the program.

Physicians are key team members in a dual diagnosis program. In order to treat a client with coexisting psychiatric and substance abuse problems effectively, it is imperative to have a psychiatrist who is comfortable with a coexisting disorders model. We emphasize the need for physicians who believe that both the disease of addiction and the mental illness require comprehensive simultaneous care. We have found success in recruiting psychiatrists when we are crystal clear about our philosophy and the mission of our program, and we move quickly to intervene when prescription practices diverge from this model.

We have also found it helpful to have physicians sign a dual diagnosis treatment agreement prior to involvement in any direct inpatient care. In this agreement we ask physicians to agree to the following regarding the subject patients:

- No use of addictive substances after detox without prior approval of the medical director and/or clinical director or equivalent.
- Mandatory attendance of patients at AA or NA meetings both during treatment and as part of the discharge plan.
- Psychological evaluations of all patients treated to ensure a comprehensive assessment.
- Mandatory patient attendance in family therapy.
- No discharge of a patient until aftercare plans are complete.
- Adherence to all rules of the program regarding urine drug screens, passes, visitation rules, level system (specifying privileges), and so on.

We have the same expectations where appropriate in outpatient programs.

We have found that by making clear from the start all of our program expectations we create a more congenial atmosphere among treatment team members. Those individuals who tend to be uncomfortable with the treatment agreement have turned out to have a difficult time working with the rest of the treatment team. Therefore, the agreement serves two purposes: (1) it screens out anyone who is adamantly opposed to our philosophy; and (2) it makes clear our philosophy and mission to all team members prior to specific conflicts arising and provides a basis for resolving conflicts that do arise.

We would love to tell you that we have little difficulty in finding open-minded individuals with fantastic clinical skills who have training and experience in working with psychiatric problems as well as with chemical dependency problems—but unfortunately that is not the case. We have found that we can just as easily train a mental health professional to do chemical dependency counseling as we can train a chemical dependency counselor to work with psychiatric patients. We do prefer a recovering professional with experiential knowledge of recovery. However, the key issue is the individual and his/her attitude. It is important to find individuals who, like the physician, can accept the concept of coexisting disorders and simultaneous treatment.

We have found it particularly effective to have both recovering and nonrecovering individuals and both chemical dependency counselors and mental health clinicians on the staff to maintain a balance of approaches and to help cross-train one another. Staff members who do not believe in both the disease process of the psychiatric disorder and the disease process of the addiction tend to experience conflict with other team members and to be less effective in their clinical care of a dually diagnosed client. At a minimum, they are not helpful to the overall recovery of the client. At worst, they engender splits and conflicts among other treatment team members and the patient, and thus they may significantly undermine the recovery of the client.

Ongoing training and supervision are essential to the professional growth of all clinicians, helping them to avoid "relapses" back into ongoing, rigid primary–secondary thinking and to cope better with the special demands of working with clients with dual disorders. In training new staff, we find it helpful to have them read this book. We also strongly encourage our staff to attend several AA/NA meetings and to become familiar with the self-help groups in their locality. We also hold frequent in-services on mental health and chemical dependency issues and their interaction. We have both group and individual supervision weekly. We also have a special monthly supervision session for those with a mental health background to learn from a chemical dependency treatment person, and vice versa.

Readers may also find helpful the report of the Center for Mental Health Services Managed Care Initiative: Clinical Standards and Workforce Competencies Project (Minkoff & Rossi, 1998) useful in implementing or revising programs.

MANAGED HEALTH CARE

Managed health care in general seeks the least expensive (typically least intensive and restrictive) care required by the severity of clients' illnesses and flexible, clinically driven, individualized treatment plans provided by appropriately credentialed personnel (Mee-Lee, 1994). The goal is cost-effective treatment. Managed care overall has increased, to good effect, the accountability of treatment providers in the chemical dependency and mental health fields. At the same time, our experience has been that the efforts at cost containment have led, ironically, to an increase in our own administrative overhead. Some reviews are very perfunctory and of minimal import. Others, however, are extremely burdensome in terms of high levels of paperwork or of very frequent reviews, with all the phone tag and the need to track review status that this entails. Couple this with reimbursement rates that have been negotiated down and essentially frozen for the past decade and we find that we are continually having to work harder for less. At some point, this productivity crunch cannot continue.

Specific issues arise with regard to clients with dual disorders. Most insurances have separate benefits for chemical dependency and mental health treatment, and their payment and authorization systems are separately tracked. Many times reviewers get confused when we request chemical dependency treatment and a psychiatric medication evaluation and then have to go through their supervisors to get exceptions. This delay can be frustrating and confusing to all parties. At the same time, when we have carefully explained the situation, most reviewers are accommodating. Especially with acute psychiatric symptoms, we have even found that authorizations are more easily obtained than with single diagnosis alcoholics/addicts. Other things being equal, we tend to use the chemical dependency benefit first if we have the option of tapping both benefits. These benefits are sometimes more generous than the mental health ones. Probably the most frustrating issue is when an insurance company or managed health care contract only allows the larger of both benefits to be tapped. This fails to take into account the synergistic problems of dually disordered clients and, most especially, the need for longer treatments. In these cases we have resorted to a number of stratagems. We have sought out grants for treating dually diagnosed clients without resources. We also use group therapy more because it generally costs less than individual treatment. Finally, we have gone to discounted rates for clients who can pay cash.

Despite the increasingly widespread image of managed health care as a big bad bogeyman, public sources of funding, in our experience, are even more rigid than health maintenance organizations (HMOs) about paying for care that addresses both disorders. In the 1990s more private treatment programs began to treat publicly treated clients. State and local governments, experimenting with the efficiency offered by nonpublic sector programs and private programs, have sought other sources of funding as insurance money funds decreased. However, even though private programs have designed information systems to meet the requirements of insurance and managed health care, such programs have not been accustomed to the lengthy bureaucratic paperwork required by government funding sources. In addition, directors of public agencies typically have had no clinical responsibilities, and their primary responsibilities often just included meetings with other directors for planning and networking. Private agencies, in contrast, have had to "trim the fat" to compete in the managed health care market and have often had directors who were required to do much more than simply direct and manage the bureaucracy. Private agencies also have had to pay higher salaries than in public agencies to attract the credentialed clinicians required by managed health care and have had to choose between data collection and reporting and client care.

Finally, multiple parties of the government, at different federal, state, and county levels have typically set client eligibility criteria. Often these criteria have been either too rigid or too vague, without one central authority to make quick decisions about a particular client. As a result, clinicians are not always certain whether their client is eligible for funding. With managed care, however, there is someone in authority who can make prompt decisions about a client and can determine whether clients are eligible for funds for psychiatric evaluation and medication.

Some authors have expressed the hope that managed health care will ultimately provide the push necessary to reunite treatment systems in the name of cost-effective treatment (Osher & Drake, 1996). Only time will tell.

CHAPTER 4

Assessing Chemical Dependency in the Dually Diagnosed Client

A Bar
A bar to heaven,
A door to hell,
Whoever named it,
Named it well.
    —ANONYMOUS

In earlier chapters we discussed how care providers frequently serve clients with dual diagnoses. In this chapter we elaborate some simple principles and techniques for assessing the chemical dependency half of the equation. The discussion first focuses on basic principles of identifying symptoms of chemical dependency in general. We then examine the application of these principles to dually diagnosed persons.

THE QUALITY ASPECT

There is no agreed-upon professional standard for assessing substance use disorders. All procedures have their strengths and limitations. Authors typically suggest using two or more methods to enhance accuracy, both with "alcoholic-only" and dual diagnosis clients (Drake, Rosenberg, & Mueser, 1996). Most clinicians rely on interviews and urine drug screens.

The clinician attempting to interview someone and assess whether that person is chemically dependent needs to keep in mind several important concepts. It is very tempting to jump right in and start asking questions regarding the kind and amount of drugs and alcohol used. However, this should not be the main thrust of the assessment. Remember that *quantity* of use is not the basis for a diagnosis of chemical dependency. Rather, *quality* of use is the prime consideration. Another way to phrase the key issue is this: it is *not* how much, or how often, but *what happens* when this person uses chemicals that matters most.

LOSS OF CONTROL

The essential factor in making an accurate assessment of chemical dependency, aside from physical dependence as demonstrated by tolerance and withdrawal symptoms, is *loss of control.* Is there an indication that the individual has been unsuccessful in controlling the use of drugs and alcohol? Specifics to look for when evaluating for loss of control are:

1. Did the person drink or use more than planned?
2. Does the individual have rules about his/her use of chemicals (such as "I'll only drink wine," "I'll only drink after 5:00 P.M.," "I'll never drink alone," "I can only have one drink per hour")?
3. Does the individual ever break or dismiss his/her own rules about drinking or using?
4. Has the individual tried to control his/her drinking/using or tried to control situations where he/she misbehaves when drinking and using? Was he/she successful in controlling his/her use of chemicals or did he/she eventually lose control of consumption or behaviors when imbibing, inhaling, and so on? Did he/she vow to stop and not do this, or stop only for a short time?

Loss of control need not be each and every time the person uses for there to be a problem. Persons in the early or middle stages of chemical dependency may lose control only occasionally to start. The difficulty for individuals is that they cannot predict on what occasions they will lose control of their drinking or using and what negative life consequences might follow their unsuccessful attempts to control the uncontrollable. Questions about what happened during past efforts to cut down or quit also help to identify the presence of withdrawal symptoms and issues of loss of control as well as factors influencing motivation and relapse.

NEGATIVE CONSEQUENCES

Negative consequences related to drinking and using behavior are a strong indicator that individuals are in the throes of addiction. Father Joseph Martin, a famous priest in the field of addiction, describes the criteria for identifying alcoholism simply as "What causes problems is a problem." If drinking and drugging behavior are causing problems in someone's life and the individual keeps drinking and using drugs in spite of these problems, then that person has a problem with drugs and alcohol.

It is also important that an evaluator look at different areas of life function and any problems in these areas. Frequently, these problems are a result of substance abuse. Sometimes these functional impairments are the smoke that indicates the fire of problematic chemical use—even before there is any specific or detailed information about chemical use. The evaluator should remember that, owing to denial, the client is unlikely to admit to a direct causal relationship between his/her drinking and his/her thorniest problems. (We discuss denial in detail later in this chapter.)

Social and Recreational Problems

Social problems can be an early indicator of a drug or alcohol problem. Look for things like the following:

1. A change in friends (no longer associating with nonabusers)
2. Feeling uncomfortable in settings where no alcohol is served nor drugs available
3. Friends and family complaining about the use of the chemical or the behavior associated with substance abuse
4. An inability to attend social gatherings without a "prefunction" (drugs or alcohol used prior to the function)
5. Feeling guilty over social behavior when drinking or using
6. Behavior when drinking or using that is not consistent with the value system of the individual
7. Sexual acting out when drinking or using—for example, promiscuity, having detrimental affairs, unusual sexual behavior, group sex, prostitution, and so on
8. No continuing interest in previously valued hobbies, sports, clubs, and the like
9. Drinking and using in secret or alone

Legal Problems

Many substance abusers find themselves with a host of legal problems. A history of any of the following may be an indicator of a drug or alcohol problem:

1. Arrest for driving under the influence
2. Assault (nonfelony)
3. Burglary

4. Shoplifting
5. Driving with a suspended license
6. Reckless driving
7. "Solicitation" (prostitution)
8. Breaking and entering
9. Drug trafficking or distribution

Adolescents typically have their own set of legal problems. These include the following:

1. Minor in possession (of drugs)
2. Burglary
3. Vandalism
4. Prostitution
5. Breaking and entering
6. Grand theft auto
7. Criminal mischief
8. Runaway, truancy, other status (noncriminal) offenses

Family Problems

Family conflict is an indicator of a drug and alcohol problem. Some theorists have put the cart before the horse in always assuming that persons drink and use chemicals because of family conflict. In reality, much of the family conflict can very often be a result of substance abuse. In other cases abuse or dependence exacerbates existing conflict. Things to look for are:

1. An increase in family conflict (not only with the substance abuser but also among other non-drug-abusing family members) around such things as failure to live up to expectations regarding work, school, family life, and disregard of family rules
2. Sexual problems with the spouse
3. Avoiding contact with family members
4. Physical illness, depression, or the acting out of other family members
5. Runaway or being ejected from the home
6. Neglect of children, violence, sexual assault

Besides negative consequences related directly to the client's substance use, other aspects of the family need to be assessed. Information about a family history of problems with substances can yield information on genetic risk factors (as well as for such issues as childhood trauma). Knowledge of the current chemical use of family members and their attitudes toward the client's use and toward the possibility of the client's entry into sobriety are important in assessing the level of support for his/ her changing.

Medical Problems

There are many medical problems that are a direct result of substance abuse, some of which are very common to alcoholics and addicts. Medical concerns that are often indicators of substance abuse include the following:

1. Sleep disturbances
2. Gastritis
3. Intestinal difficulties
4. Hepatitis
5. Unwanted pregnancy
6. Eating disorders
7. Stress-exacerbated illnesses, including mouth ulcers and migraine headaches
8. Vague complaints, complaints of general malaise
9. Malnutrition
10. Stomach ulcers
11. Emphysema
12. Accidents, falls
13. Suicide attempts
14. Sexual disorders
15. Hypertension
16. Heart disease, stroke
17. Diabetes or hypoglycemia
18. HIV, AIDS
19. Rape
20. Heart dysrhythmias
21. Skin infections

Employment

For gainfully employed substance abusers, their jobs are often the last area to be affected by drug or alcohol abuse. Persons with substance use disorders frequently hold up their job as an example of how drinking or using is not a problem. In addition, the income from employment is needed to continue providing funds for procuring alcohol and/or drugs.

Indicators in the workplace that an individual may have a drug and/or alcohol problem include the following:

1. Difficulty in getting along with coworkers
2. Frequent medical problems and use of sick time
3. Oversensitivity to feedback or criticism by one's supervisor(s)
4. Monday or Friday tardiness or absenteeism
5. Inconsistent performance
6. Tardiness in general
7. Labile, moody behavior

Adolescents, or those otherwise in school, can exhibit such problems as these:

1. Academic underachievement
2. Dropping out of school or expulsion
3. Suspension for fighting, a negative attitude, or possession of contraband
4. Truancy
5. Isolation
6. Amotivational syndrome (apathy)
7. A sudden change of friends
8. Sleeping during class
9. A negative attitude toward authority figures
10. A labile mood

THE QUANTITY ASPECT

Loss of control and negative consequences are the cardinal signs of chemical dependency, encompassing the quality aspect. Nonetheless, information about the kinds, quantities, frequency, and history of substance use is also important. Data on first regular use (defined as once a week or more) can provide a baseline for determining progression. While most clients have a preferred substance, the available data indicate that polysubstance dependence is very common. Not only using more and more of a given chemical, but also using more and more of different kinds of chemicals, is indicative of progression, as well. Specific information about quantities can help to determine the development of tolerance. In addition, data about last use and use during the preceding week are particularly important in determining current intoxication and in assessing the need for medical detoxification.

WITHDRAWAL AND MEDICAL ISSUES

The signs and symptoms of withdrawal are usually the reverse of the direct pharmacological effects of the drug. Alcohol, for example, usually reduces anxiety and causes sedation, and in large quantities can produce sleep, coma, and death. For persons physically dependent on alcohol, stopping its intake produces anxiety, agitation, nausea and vomiting, tremor, sweats, insomnia, headache, hallucinations, disorientation, and seizures. Withdrawal from some chemicals such as alcohol, barbiturates, and the benzodiazepines can be life-threatening. Signs and symptoms of acute alcohol withdrawal generally begin 6–24 hours after the last drink. With certain barbiturates and benzodiazepines, withdrawal symptoms peak 5 to 8 days after the last dose but can occur as late as two weeks afterward. Opioid and stimulant withdrawal is usually evident after 8 to 12 hours. Withdrawal from these substances is not usually life-threatening per se but is extremely distressful, and there is the risk of suicide, especially with the "crash" of stimulant withdrawal. A federally sponsored Treatment Improvement Protocol (Wesson, 1995) is a comprehensive overview of issues regarding withdrawal and detoxification issues.

Severinghaus and Kinney (1996) enumerate certain conditions that indicate the need for immediate medical evaluation or for nonemergent (less time-sensitive) evaluation. Those indicating a need for immediate medical attention include the following:

1. Recent substance intake at levels that risk developing toxicity, poisoning, or organ damage even if the client is asymptomatic
2. Ingestion of unknown quantities and substances
3. Confusion or delirium
4. Tachycardia (heart rate >110 bpm)
5. History of evidence of physical trauma, especially head trauma
6. Client semiconscious and able to be roused but falls asleep when stimulus removed
7. History of a difficult withdrawal
8. Severe tremors
9. Hallucinations or marked paranoia
10. Severe agitation
11. Fever
12. Polysubstance dependence
13. Seizures or a history of seizures
14. Rapid intake of chemicals

Conditions indicating a need for nonemergent medical evaluation include:

1. Recent history of bleeding
2. No recent medical evaluation (for clients with an extended history of heavy alcohol or drug use)
3. Complaints of not feeling well
4. History of chronic medical conditions for which clients are not getting care

Providers who are not medical personnel should have easy access to medical consultation and back-up because of these kinds of medical issues.

OTHER IMPORTANT INFORMATION

Clinicians should attempt to assess other information as part of a quality chemical use assessment. This assessment should include the history of use over time; clients' expectations regarding use and treatment; attendance at self-help groups and treatment episodes; periods of abstinence; triggers for relapses; the current motivation for treatment; and social support for sobriety versus pressure for use. Clinicians can use these data to formulate a treatment plan.

DENIAL

Human beings tend to avoid situations that cause conflict or emotional stress. All of us are familiar with the fight-or-flight response. Our instinct is to either engage in battle or run away when faced with a threatening situation. Addiction is a primary urge—that is, using the substance is more important to the impaired user than food, shelter, love, or money. When the primary focus of your life is threatened, the natural fight-or-flight instinct takes over. People do not usually club to death those who threaten their chemical use. Instead, they develop mental defenses that protect them *psychologically* from harm. A major defense is *denial.*

There are two forms of denial. One involves conscious lying, and the others, subconscious self-delusion. In the first form of denial one is aware of the lying behavior. For example, Jane says to Paul, "You've been drinking," after smelling alcohol on his breath. Paul, who realizes Jane smells the five beers he just drank, tries to cover up the fact with a lie and says, "No, you are mistaken." Paul is "denying" that he drank, but he is aware that he is not being truthful. In the second situation (illustrating subconscious self-delusion), Jane says to Paul, "You act like you're drunk again. I think you're an alcoholic!" Upon hearing this, Paul feels that his ability to drink is threatened. If he really believes what Jane says, then he would have to change his behavior, which would be extremely difficult for him. Paul's psychological defenses come to the rescue. He quickly justifies his behavior, then switches to blaming Jane by responding, "Who wouldn't drink, with a nagging wife like you? Besides, you think everybody is an alcoholic!" Paul is not consciously aware that he is "in denial." His rationalization (Jane's nagging) becomes the way he flees from the danger threatening his primary urge to drink.

THINKING ERRORS

There are many "mistakes" in thinking that alcoholics/addicts develop in order to protect their drinking and/or using. Whenever the chemically dependent person engages in behavior that is against his/her own value system, he/she is forced to either (1) change the behavior or (2) change the way he/she thinks about the behavior. As the disease of addiction progresses, so do the mistakes or errors in thinking made by the alcoholic. Stanton Samenow, PhD, in his work with sociopaths (Samenow, 1984), developed a list of "thinking errors" commonly seen in clients with antisocial personality disorder. We have adapted Dr. Samenow's list for our work with alcoholics and addicts. We do not believe that alcoholics and addicts are criminals but merely that they develop a style of thinking embodying typical antisocial attitudes as part of their denial system. The next section presents a list of common thinking errors frequently resorted to by both criminals and alcoholics. All of these thinking errors are forms of denial. The thinking errors of the alcoholic disappear once the alcoholic enters sobriety.

Alcoholic/Antisocial Thinking Errors

1. *Excuse making.* Alcoholics make excuses for anything and everything. Whenever held accountable for drinking or using behavior, alcoholics often give excuses (however lame they might be). Excuses are a means of finding reasons to justify their behavior.

EXAMPLE: "I drink because I'm depressed" or "I drink because my wife doesn't understand me."

2. *Blaming.* Blaming is an excuse not to solve a problem, and alcoholics use blaming to excuse their behavior and build up resentment toward someone else for "causing" whatever has happened.

EXAMPLE: "I couldn't do it because he got in my way"; "The trouble with you is you're always looking at me in a critical way"; "My wife nags me too much about my drinking."

Blaming permits the buildup of resentments and gets the focus off the alcoholic and onto others.

3. *Redefining*. Redefining is shifting the focus of an issue to avoid solving a problem.

> EXAMPLE: Question: "Why did you violate your abstinence contract by drinking?"
>
> Answer: "I feel the language in the contract was too wordy and confusing."

Alcoholics use redefining to get the focus off the subject in question. Redefining also indicates ineffective thinking, of not dealing with the problem at hand.

4. *Superoptimism.* "I think, therefore it is." The superoptimistic person decides that, because he wants something to be a certain way, or thinks it will be a certain way, therefore it is or will be that particular way. This superoptimistic attitude—however fanciful and unrealistic—permits a person to function according to what he/she wants rather than in concert with the facts of the situation.

> EXAMPLE: Alcoholics sometimes really believe that they can stop drinking solely as a consequence of having decided to do so, with no treatment or AA support. Superoptimistic people also believe that they can be famous, popular, strong, rich, and so forth simply by wishing it and never take into account the practical steps along the way.

5. *Lying.* Lying is the most commonly known characteristic of alcoholic thinking. Most alcoholics lie in different ways at different times. They use lying to confuse, distort, and take the focus off their behavior. Lying takes three forms:

Commission: making things up that are simply not true;

Omission: saying partly what is so but leaving out major contrary portions; and

Assent: making believe that one agrees with someone else, or presenting or approving others' ideas in order to look good when, in fact, one has no intention of going along or does not really agree; "you could say that" is an example of subtle lying by assent.

6. *Making fools of others.* Alcoholics make fools of others by agreeing to do things and not following through, by saying things they do not mean, by setting others up to fight needlessly, by inviting expectations and letting people down, and in numerous other ways. By attempting to make others look ludicrous, alcoholics hope to take the focus off their own behavior.

7. *Assuming.* Alcoholics spend a great deal of time assuming they know what others think, what others feel, and what others are doing. They then use these assumptions in the service of whatever drinking or using activity or behavior they decide to engage in.

EXAMPLE: The alcoholic assumes that other people do not like him/ her. This gives him/her an excuse to blow up, be angry, or get drunk or stoned. Assuming takes place every day, and the alcoholic makes assumptions about whatever he/she wishes in order to support his/her alcoholic behavior.

8. *"I'm unique."* Alcoholics believe that they are unique and special and that no one else is like them. It therefore follows that any information that is applied to other people simply doesn't apply to them. Examples of these kinds of beliefs include "I don't need anyone, and no one understands me anyway" and "No one can tell me what to do." Alcoholics in treatment commonly believe that everyone else is an alcoholic except themselves.

9. *Ingratiating.* Alcoholics often overdo being nice to others and going out of their way to act interested in other people. They try to find out what they can get from other people, how they can manipulate them, use them, or control the situation for their own purposes. Watch out for praise from an alcoholic regarding your counseling skills!

10. *Fragmented personality.* It is not uncommon for alcoholics to, for example, attend church on Sunday, get drunk on Tuesday afternoon, and then attend church again on Wednesday evening. To alcoholics, there is no inconsistency in this behavior. They believe that they are good persons and are justified in doing whatever they do. Their acts are seen as things that they deserve to do, or get, or own, or possess, or control. They never consider such wide-ranging behaviors as inconsistent.

11. *Minimizing.* Alcoholics often minimize their behavior by talking about it in such a way that it seems insignificant. They routinely discount the significance of their behavior. You will immediately see minimizing when confronting the alcoholic about some irresponsible behavior.

EXAMPLE: "I only drank three beers, and I could have drunk a lot more, but I didn't."

12. *Vagueness.* Alcoholics are typically unclear and nonspecific to avoid being pinned down on any particular issue. They use words and phrases that are lacking in detail. In this way they can look good to others but not commit themselves to anything specific.

EXAMPLE: Vague words include phrases such as: "I more or less think so"; "I guess"; "probably"; "maybe"; "I might"; "I'm not sure about"; and "I smoke pot occasionally."

13. *Anger.* Anger is a primary emotion for the alcoholic. Alcoholics use the anger to control others or to leverage their power in a situation. Alcoholics have unrealistic expectations about the people in their world and control others through aggression, physical or verbal attacks, criticism, or in any other way that immobilizes others, and better enables them to control the situation.

14. *Power plays.* Alcoholics use power plays whenever they aren't getting their way in a situation. These include such things as walking out of a room during a disagreement, not completing a job that he/she agrees to do, refusing to listen or hear what someone else has to say, and organizing people to be angry at others in support.

15. *Victim playing.* This is a major role that alcoholics can take. The underlying issues are aggression and power plays. However, alcoholics act as though they are unable to solve problems or do anything for themselves. Alcoholics often whine, shuffle, look woebegone and helpless, and act as if they are too stupid to do anything for themselves. The alcoholics' belief is that if they do not get whatever they want then they are a victim. Victim playing elicits constructive criticism, rescue, or enabling behavior from those around them while it sidesteps responsibility for alcoholics' own behavior.

16. *Drama/excitement.* Because alcoholics do not live a real life in the sense of getting their needs met directly, they often create unnecessary drama and excitement whenever feasible. Excitement is a distraction and keeps the focus off alcoholics' own behavior and their drinking.

17. *Closed channel.* Alcoholics are secretive and often closed-minded. Alcoholics need to protect their drinking and using lifestyle. Therefore, when confronted with data about their behavior, they are closed-minded and refuse to acknowledge the input, as it might jeopardize their continued drinking.

18. *Image.* The alcoholic's image of him/herself is important to maintain. Even a late-stage skid-row alcoholic will express concern at being seen at an AA meeting.

19. *Grandiosity.* Grandiosity is minimizing or maximizing the significance of an issue, and it is used to justify not solving a problem.

EXAMPLE: "I've spilled more booze than you drank"; "I can drink everyone under the table and drive them all home, so I'm not an alcoholic."

20. *Intellectualizing.* Using academic, abstract, or theoretical discussions to avoid dealing with feelings or the real issues.

When trying to assess an individual, it is important to recognize that person's denial system for what it is. It is not reasonable to assume that alcoholics or addicts are necessarily going to be open and honest with us about their use of chemicals. This is especially true if clients face mandatory treatment, revocation of probation, loss of housing, or other negative consequences. If treatment is one consequence, we are threatening their primary need to drink and use. Clients are often unable to be honest with us (or with themselves) prior to treatment. However, when interviewing a client, if you notice a client's heavy indulgence in "thinking errors" when discussing his/her chemical use, this in itself may be an indication of a substance abuse problem. Dually diagnosed clients will normally evidence obvious thinking errors when they are using chemicals. Even individuals suffering from psychotic symptoms opt for denial in their response to questions about chemical use. Given the prevalence of denial, professionals have looked at additional ways to increase the accuracy of assessments.

INTERVIEWING STRATEGIES

Professionals have outlined interview guidelines that seem to be helpful in increasing the accuracy of clients' self-report (O'Connor, 1996; Sobell, Toneatto, & Sobell, 1994; Miller & Rollnick, 1991; Babor, Brown, & DelBoca, 1990). These include the following:

1. Use an open-ended format for questions (questions that begin with what, when, etc., and not questions that can be answered simply yes or no) and make questions specific and factual.
2. Recognize vague, qualified answers and be gently persistent in getting specifics.
3. Use periodic summaries and solicit clients' feedback about them.
4. Roll with resistance and avoid argumentation and confrontation.
5. Express empathy through reflective listening, reflecting both sides of the ambivalence (on one hand, on the other), and use Socratic questioning.
6. Affirm clients through sincere compliments.
7. Adopt a matter-of-fact approach and avoid taking defensiveness personally.
8. Avoid discussion of rationalizations.
9. Move only very slowly to introduce the label of alcoholic or addict.
10. Check to see if clients understand such terms as blackouts, tolerance, etc.
11. Use standardized tests to increase accuracy and to give objective feedback.
12. Make extensive use of instructions to orient clients to the purposes and procedures of the interview.
13. Start with relatively neutral questions and ask sensitive questions later on.
14. Elicit a commitment to honesty at the beginning of the interview.
15. Ask about past or lifetime behavior first, then go to current behavior.
16. Inform clients that other sources of information will also be used.
17. Avoid interviewing an intoxicated individual.

We also find it instructive to note clients' reactions to a request for an abstinence contract, releases of information to significant others, or for a "preventative" trial of Antabuse (taking it before the weekend, for example, to prevent a relapse and "just in case"). A sudden surge in defensiveness to such requests can be very instructive and point to possible substance use problems.

COLLATERAL CONTACTS

We cannot emphasize enough the need for collateral data. You *must* have information from sources other than the clients' self-report. Obtaining collateral data is an excellent way to complement the interview with the client in assessing a client for chemical dependency. Given the self-deception and denial of substance abusers, you cannot rely exclusively on data provided to you by these individuals. You can sometimes ferret out the facts, but do not put too much stock in the alcoholic's or addict's explanation of the situation. Family members, employers, court workers, physicians, and friends can all be excellent sources of information. Remember, however, that they too may suffer from denial, stemming either from their own need to deny the problem or from having listened too often to the excuses and explanations made by the chemically dependent person. Or they may not have sufficient contact with clients to really qualify as collateral with useful information.

Keep your questions to these people factually based. Ask, for example, "How many days a month is Paul calling in sick?" or "Has Paul ever been arrested before?" We should not expect others to have attributed specific behavior to the use of chemicals. Asking such questions as "Do you think Paul's an alcoholic?" may prove very unproductive. This and most of the other interview strategies just outlined are relevant to interviewing collateral contacts. In our experience, clients who refuse to give releases of information for a collateral contact are generally attempting to control the situation, and we deal with this issue directly before proceeding further with the assessment and any treatment.

OTHER METHODS OF EVALUATING CHEMICAL USE AND DEPENDENCY
Lab Procedures

Are there other, less fallible, methods of assessing chemical use and dependency, ones easily accessible to most service providers?

Most psychoactive substances, with the exception of LSD and alcohol, can be detected up to 48–72 hours in urine. Breath analysis or urinalysis is only sensitive to alcohol used in the preceding 12–24 hours. Because of this time constraint, breath analysis or urinalysis typically has limited use in normal outpatient settings. LSD and inhalants require costly and specialized procedures for analysis. Chronic pot smokers will evidence THC (tetrahydro cannibinol) in the urine for as long as 30 days or more. Urinalysis does have the advantage of being able to detect both alcohol and other drugs. This is an important consideration for the dually disordered population, with its high rates of polysubstance abuse and use of street drugs sold as one substance but containing mixtures of other substances. The lab can also provide not only qualitative but quantitative levels. This is helpful with the cannabis users who claim no recent use. Decreasing nanogram levels of THC can confirm this and provide a way to monitor progress. The increasing sophistication of certified laboratory procedures can detect attempts to fake negative urinalyses and determine whether over-the-counter cold remedies could account for a positive urinalysis for stimulants. Procedures for informed consent and for safeguarding clients' privacy and dignity can minimize the invasiveness of urinalyses. We have criteria for deciding which clients are to have monitored urinalyses, and have two same-sex staff members do the monitoring. We have found that matter-of-fact explanations that urinanalyses are routine and that refusal to give a urine sample is considered a positive urinalysis for substances gives us a high rate of compliance. To protests that "You don't trust me!" we simply respond that we trust the client, we just don't trust the disease.

Many professionals and certainly the public tend to see urine testing as the gold standard for assessing clients' chemical use. Yet, in addition to some of the limitations outlined above, urine tests, while generally accurate, do sometimes yield false positives and negatives (Maisto, McKay, & Connors, 1990). The public's faith in their accuracy may make urine tests most useful as a prompt to honesty and only secondarily useful as a foolproof assistance to accurate diagnosis.

Other physical tests are possible, but all have limitations (Maisto et al., 1990). Hair analysis can detect drug use over several years and is highly accurate but also very expensive. Saliva dipstick tests have rates of false positives and negatives that are higher than urinalysis, and drugs are retained for shorter periods in saliva than urine, decreasing the time period for detection. Acute liver function tests appear to be able to assess alcohol consumption over time periods longer than 24 hours, but a number of other factors that also influence liver function can make the interpretation of findings problematic. High current blood levels of a psychoactive substance without signs of intoxication suggest tolerance.

This implies chronic use of that substance or ones from the same family (cross-tolerance). A tolerance challenge is another assessment method. Administering phenobarbital, for example, with no subsequent signs of intoxication suggests chronic use of sedatives, hypnotics, or anxiolytics. Similarly, the administration of an opiate blocker such as naloxone will precipitate an acute withdrawal reaction in a person dependent on opiates. Readers can consult with medical personnel or the staff of their local medical laboratory for additional information about these tests. The problem with these tests is that they require a hospital setting, medical personnel, expensive procedures, and informed consent except in emergency situations.

Questionnaires

A number of questionnaires exist that inquire directly about chemical use and use-related behavior. The Michigan Alcoholism Screening Test is a well-known inventory (Seyler, 1971). The problem is that clients can fake answers to inventories. The developers of these inventories also had adults in mind when designing them. However, we do know of two self-report instruments that deal with the faking and adult-only issues. The Substance Abuse Subtle Screening Inventory (SASSI; available from the SASSI Institute, Route 2, Box 134, Springville, IN 47462) has versions for both adults and adolescents and has scales designed to detect faking. Lazowski, Miller, Boye, & Miller (1998) demonstrated a 98% accuracy rate for the SASSI-3 used with dually diagnosed inpatients. The Minnesota Multiphasic Inventory (MMPI; available from National Computer Systems, P.O. Box 1416, Minneapolis, MN 55440; 800-627-7271) has both adolescent and adult versions, updated norms, and ways of detecting faking. The validity scales of the MMPI-2 and the MMPI-A (for adolescents) and other scores derived from the test can help determine whether clients answered in a straightforward, defensive, or exaggerated manner to this test and may also indicate degree of honesty in other self-report measures (Isenhart & Silversmith, 1996). The MacAndrews Scale, designed to detect alcohol problems, does a good job with "honest" alcoholics and a fair job even with alcoholics given instructions to fake normality. The use of the Positive Malingering Scale (and a few other special scales) together with the MacAndrews does a good job of detecting alcoholics who are faking normality well (Otto, Long, Megaree, & Rosenblatt, 1988). Two other scales on the MMPI-2 for adults (the addiction potential scale and the addiction acknowledgment scale) also appear to do a good job in detecting addiction (Greene, Weed, Butcher, Arredondo, & Davis, 1992; Rouse, Butcher, & Miller, 1999). Supplementing the MacAndrews Scale found on the adult version, the adolescent version has two additional scales (substance involvement and proneness to problems) serving as indices of problematic substance use. Another advantage of using the MMPI is the information this can give on possible coexisting psychiatric disorders because the instrument has been designed to be a broad-width measure of a number of psychiatric disorders (see Chapter 5). Readers interested in using the MMPI or other inventories in their work should consult with a psychologist.

Drake, Mueser, and McHugo (1996) describe three clinicians' rating scales designed to assess and monitor substance use in persons with severe mental illness. The Alcohol Use Scale ask clinicians to rate their clients in one of five categories: abstinent, use without impairment, abuse, dependence, and dependence with institutionalization. The Drug Use Scale uses the same categories with the addition of a section to indicate drugs used. The Substance Abuse Treatment Scale asks clinicians to rate their clients as being in one of eight categories of recovery: preengagement, engagement, early persuasion, late persuasion, early active treatment, late active treatment, relapse prevention, and remission, or recovery. Reliability and validity are excellent. As far as we know, these are the only scales specifically designed for dually diagnosed clients. Unfortunately, as the authors point out, these questionnaires do not serve as the basis for a comprehensive evaluation. They also assume that the data available on clients are accurate.

More Information on the Validity of Self-Reports and Other Assessment Techniques

The validity of self-reports for substance abusers in general appears to vary considerably, depending mainly on the circumstances under which the data are collected (Babor et al., 1990). When substance abusers are alcohol- and drug-free, are interviewed in clinical or research settings, and are given assurances of confidentiality, the data would appear to be valid (Sobell et al., 1994). Conversely, the accuracy of self-reports appears to decrease when clients are not drug-free, for example. We have also seen an interesting phenomenon where clients coming to our clinic for assessment and treatment of mental health problems are quite honest about their use of substances until they discover that we also treat drug and alcohol problems. These clients deny that the two six-packs a night Thursday through Sunday has anything to do with their depression. Validity of collaterals' information who have high contact with clients appears to be good, but there is also some tendency for collaterals to underestimate clients' drug and alcohol use (Sobel et al., 1994).

Similar complexity appears to hold for clients with dual disorders. Studies of dually diagnosed persons suffering from schizophrenia have found underreporting of drug use in an emergency room setting and at a medication clinic (Stone, Greenstein, Gamble, & Mclellan, 1993; Shaner et al., 1993). On the other hand, in a study of dually diagnosed outpatients with bipolar or posttraumatic stress disorder, Weiss, Najavits, et al. (1998) found a high rate of agreement between self-reports of substance use and supervised urine samples. They attributed the high levels of agreement to the fact that their subjects were already in treatment, data were collected repeatedly over time, urine samples were collected with patients' prior knowledge, were well known to staff, and entailed no negative consequences, thus encouraging honest self-reporting. One study of substance abuse in psychiatric inpatients showed that substance abuse diagnoses doubled after assessment with standardized interviews (Lyons & McGovern, 1989), and another concluded that urine toxicology analyses and admission and discharge diagnoses were significantly less accurate in diagnosing a substance use disorder than was the SCID-P, a structured clinical interview tied to DSM-III-R (American Psychiatric Association, 1987). (Albanese, Barter, Bruno, Morgenbessen, & Schatzberg, 1994). Another study examined the utility of the Addiction Severity Index (a well-known, reliable, and valid structured interview for assessing domains of functioning affected by substance use) for detecting psychoactive substance use disorders among psychiatric inpatients and concluded that there was too high a "miss" level for clinical purposes (Lehman, Myers, Dixon, & Johnson, 1996). Incidentally, this same study indicated that these psychiatric inpatients uniformly experienced significant problems at even very low levels of chemical use, supporting the need for abstinence with dually diagnosed clients.

SPECIAL CONSIDERATION FOR DUALLY DIAGNOSED CLIENTS

The first and obvious point to remember is to be sure to assess for substance use issues. As we have seen, prevalence is high in this population, as are failures to detect the problem (Drake, Rosenberg, & Mueser, 1996).

In attempting to apply traditional chemical dependency assessment criteria to clients with dual disorders there are special considerations that the evaluator needs to take into account. In the pattern of their substance abuse, dually diagnosed clients bear several similarities to "alcoholic-only" clients, including the following:

1. *Loss of control.* This symptom of chemical dependency is often clear in dually diagnosed clients. Related problems that clients experience because of the psychiatric problem (such as poor impulse control) are also heightened greatly with chemical use.

2. *Negative consequences of use.* Remember the "what causes a problem is a problem" definition of chemical abuse and dependence. This definition is very useful in detemining whether a problem exists.

3. *Preoccupation and protecting supply.* While clients with dual disorders may show a shrinking of their world due to their illness, the organizing pull of drug use is still obvious in how and with whom they spend their time, and even how they choose to spend their disability checks. Dually diagnosed clients are also concerned about "having enough to do the job." It is common to find that they hide drugs and alcohol and have special stashes "just in case."

4. *Denial of use.* Dual diagnosed clients also tend to deny use or lie about how much or how often they use drugs or drink alcohol. These clients will manifest obvious thinking errors.

5. *Systems problems.* Many persons with a psychiatric disorder will show role dysfunction and problems with family and job. However, these persons often remain involved with family and friends and typically have routine contacts with various service providers. Dually diagnosed individuals often show heightened problems in their contacts with these systems and often have an increased frequency of contacts with the legal system.

Differences between singly and dually diagnosed clients do exist. They include the following:

1. *Blackouts.* Accurate histories are difficult to obtain from clients with dual disorders. Blackouts and memory loss are difficult to ascertain when accompanied by a coexisting psychiatric disorder marked by such symptoms as psychosis or dissociation.

2. *Tolerance.* Changes in tolerance levels are often difficult to track because of sporadic and binge use. In addition, dually diagnosed clients often are poor historians, and the evaluator will often not have valid data to assess this area.

3. *Progression of use.* Frequently clients' histories of use are difficult to assess because of the problems just described. In addition dually diagnosed clients often have limited or impaired capacity for honesty and psychological awareness.

4. *Withdrawal symptoms.* When accompanied by a coexisting psychiatric disorder, symptoms of withdrawal can be masked by the psychiatric disorder. This is especially true of subtle withdrawal symptoms such as irritability, depression, and restlessness.

5. *Double denial.* If the average alcoholic/addict has developed an elaborate denial system, then dually diagnosed individuals often suffer from twice the denial. Their world view is also impaired by mistakes in

their thinking resulting from their own mental illness. The antisocial person has a triple dose of denial. The person suffering from paranoid schizophrenia is concerned about why you want to know all this information. The individual with a major depression feels so anxious, guilty, and worthless that he/she can't bear to face "all the bad things I've done."

6. *Enhanced negative consequences at lower amounts.* Dually diagnosed clients have more negative outcomes and instability in overall functioning because of drug and alcohol abuse than individuals with only a psychiatric disorder. And this unmanageability occurs at lower amounts of the substance and generally proceeds more rapidly.

In clients with an already established psychiatric disorder, providers might want to suspect a chemical use problem when their clients demonstrate frequent episodes of escalating symptoms in the absence of obvious stressors or other potential causes. Ongoing failure to comply with the treatment recommendations despite support and structure is another clue. Chemical use will often exacerbate those symptoms and problems associated with the psychiatric disorder that the chemicals can cause in individuals even without a psychiatric disorder. Stimulants, for example, can cause psychosis in normal individuals. In our experience, the person with schizophrenia using stimulants (or marijuana) can manifest florid psychotic flareups even when taking antipsychotic medication. Alcohol can intensify acting out in psychiatric clients who already act out. Marijuana use will substantially attenuate the effectiveness of antidepressants. Alcohol and other sedatives can often substantially increase anxiety and depression in psychiatric clients (Castenada et al., 1996; Kranzler & Liebowitz, 1988). In other cases, the substance use appears to mask the psychiatric illness. Some individuals suffering from schizophrenia have reported to us, for example, that drinking helps reduce the "voices" (although others report that drinking increases "voices").

In our experience, gross noncompliance with medication regimens, failure to attend day treatment or therapy appointments, and frequent hospitalizations, especially when the client signs out against medical advice, all point to possible chemical use problems. Watch for the development of problems in other clients when a new "difficult" client enters your services, as this client may start giving drugs or even selling them to his/her "new friends."

Research findings suggest that multiple sources of data are necessary to assess the substance use disorder of dually diagnosed clients (Drake & Mercer-McFadden, 1995). Remembering that any use of alcohol or drugs is likely to be contraindicated for dually diagnosed clients also makes the evaluator's job easier.

CHAPTER 5

Assessing the Psychiatric Disorder and Planning the Appropriate Level of Care

If your eyes could only see,
The defective self inside of me.
It fills my life with fear and debris.
My mournful soul cries to be free.
—ANONYMOUS

This chapter presents a general discussion of some of the issues, principles, and procedures pertinent to establishing the psychiatric symptoms/ problems and diagnoses of clients with dual disorders. Early sections discuss such issues as functional versus diagnostic problem statements and areas that providers need to assess. Later sections review the special issues that arise in achieving differential diagnoses with dually diagnosed clients. This chapter also outlines guidelines for deciding the appropriate level of care for a given dually diagnosed client. Later chapters will describe specific signs and symptoms associated with major diagnostic categories as well as more detailed treatment plans.

FUNCTIONAL VERSUS DIFFERENTIAL DIAGNOSIS

The goal of psychiatric assessment is twofold: to achieve both *a functional and a differential diagnosis*. A functional diagnosis is a statement of the client's problems and needs, whereas a differential diagnosis is a statement of the psychiatric syndrome that is the cause of the client's symptoms and problems. Both functional and differential diagnoses drive the treatment plan. But, while they complement each other, they are also separate formulations of the client's difficulties. For example, a given client might "functionally" be suicidal and at high risk, with intent, plan, access to means, a history, and so forth. Yet, at the same time this client might suffer from one or more different or "differential" psychiatric disorders, especially the ones associated with high rates of suicidality, such as schizophrenia, major depression, and substance use disorders (Bongar, 1991). The treatment plan would then make provision for ensuring the immediate safety of the client and, depending on the probable differential diagnosis, for various medications and treatment settings.

DSM-IV (American Psychiatric Association, 1994) uses a system of five axes to record information in a way that encompasses both functional and differential diagnoses. Axis I lists major disorders, including substance use disorders. Axis II is for personality and developmental disorders. Axis III is for medical disorders. Axis IV lists stressors, including the major problem categories among members of the primary support group: social environment, educational and occupational, housing and economic, access to health care services, legal systems, and crime. Axis V allows for a numerical estimate of overall functioning termed the Global Assessment of Functioning (GAF) that uses a 0–100 rating scale, with 0 being the lowest and 100 the highest points on the scale.

PSYCHIATRIC ASSESSMENT

Adequately assessing a psychiatric patient requires a *comprehensive assessment* that includes: an examination of the client's presenting complaints; a review of the current status of his/her biological, psychological, and social systems to ascertain the client's problems and needs as well as assets and limitations; and personal and family histories, including treatment. Figure 1 depicts the intake assessment "cheat sheet" that we use at our clinic. This sheet helps to guide our interview of clients and significant others. The ASAM criteria refer to the standards for determining the level of care for clients with substance use disorders developed by the American Society of Addiction Medicine (Readers will find an expanded explanation of the ASAM criteria under "Treatment Decisions" later in this chapter.)

A good *history* is an absolute necessity for establishing the differential diagnosis. Never diagnose using information based only on the client's presentation at the time of assessment. Without a good history to establish the duration and probable cause of the disorder, grave errors are possible. As with assessment of substance use, *collateral contact* is important as well. Individuals suffering from psychiatric disorders are often poor historians and are prone to systematic biases in their world view. This is particularly important for persons with psychotic symptoms, organic mental disorders and personality disorders.

FIGURE 1. Client Intake Tool

PRESENTING PROBLEMS: Referral source; why here; brief history of problems; factors leading to admission now; persons accompanying; external mandates, etc.; client's goals, wishes, fears, concerns

MENTAL STATUS: Appearance and grooming; attitude toward interviewer; reliability of information; orientation; concentration, attention; recent/remote memory; affect, mood; speech process, volume, content; thought process and content; insight/judgment; notable or unusual behavior

ALCOHOL/DRUG/TOBACCO: Type, amount, frequency; methods of administration; history of use, including first, peak, and last use; negative consequences of use, including medical, legal, school/work, family, personal areas; attempts to change pattern, stop, cut down; progression; personality changes; preoccupation(s); blackouts, withdrawal, tolerance; treatment/support group history, longest time sober, triggers for relapse

MENTAL HEALTH: Psychological/psychiatric problems and history; affective, anxiety, psychotic, explosive, trauma/dissociative, and, if indicated, organic disorders such as motor vehicle accident injury; specifically address self/other harm, past and present, and impulsiveness; treatment/support group history; response to medication; triggers for relapse

FAMILY: Marital, child, other family members, status; family history, past and present, of alcohol and drugs use, mental health issues; divorce/custody issues, significant deaths, moves

SOCIAL: Social support system, including quality, quantity, and risk issues; whether person is asking/getting support; attitudes toward chemical use, mental health problems

ETHNIC/LANGUAGE: Ethnic, cultural identification, language if an issue

RELIGIOUS: Church affiliations, spiritual beliefs, participation

EDUCATIONAL: Educational attainment/goals, history of learning disabilities and special education, current school problems if relevant

VOCATIONAL: If applicable, current employment status/future goals, job problems and their history

MILITARY: If applicable, military status, history

FINANCIAL: Income sources and any financial difficulties and their history, living arrangements if problematic

LEGAL: Legal issues, past and present, especially criminal charges, jail time, probation; if indicated, criminal activity committed but not detected or prosecuted

MEDICAL: Current physical health conditions, medications, planned/possible medical procedures; last physical; if indicated, risk of withdrawal and infectious disease risk; if indicated, pregnancy status, risk

NUTRITIONAL: Weight loss/gain, adequacy of intake, anorexia/bulimia

FIGURE 1. (*continued*)

DEVELOPMENTAL HISTORY: Pregnancy/birth complications, developmental milestones achieved on time

DIAGNOSTIC IMPRESSION: Axis I for major disorders; Axis II for personality and developmental disorders; Axis III for medical disorders; Axis IV for stressors; Axis V for GAF 0–100 rating; Axis IV problem categories include primary support group, social environment, educational and occupational, housing and economic, access to health care service, legal system, crime

GAF Ratings

100   Superior functioning in wide range of activities
90   Absent or minimal symptoms
80   If symptoms, transient and expectable reactions to psychosocial stressors
70   Some mild symptoms or some difficulty in social functioning
60   Moderate symptoms or difficulty in functioning
50   Serious symptoms or impairment
40   Some impairment in reality testing or major impairment in several areas
30   Behavior is considerably influenced by delusions or hallucinations or serious impairment in communication or judgment or inability to function in almost all areas
20   Some danger of hurting self or others or sometimes fails to maintain minimal self-care or gross impairment in communication
10   Persistent danger of severely hurting self or others or persistently poor self-care or serious suicidal act with clear expectation of death

PROBLEM LIST: The issues that will be the focus of treatment, with at least one problem per Axis I diagnosis; do not list a limitation as a problem

STRENGTHS/LIMITATIONS: Factors facilitating or hindering implementation of the treatment plan; mention at least one of each per client; includes intelligence, personality, insight, motivation, social support, spiritual beliefs against suicide, etc.

SUMMARY: Justification of the DSM-IV, Axis I diagnoses, citing specific symptoms meeting the diagnostic criteria; a prognostic statement; a summary of the treatment plan; and a rationale for the suggested level of treatment; the rationale specifically addresses the seven ASAM dimensions for alcohol and drug use and equivalent areas for mental health

ASAM CRITERIA LEVEL I OUTPATIENT AND LEVEL II INTENSIVE OUTPATIENT

1. *Detox/withdrawal*
   I. No risk of withdrawal
   II. Minimal risk or manageable on outpatient basis

2. *Physical health*
   I. and II. No health problems *or* stable and can be coordinated with primary care physician/primary caregivers

3. *Emotional/behavioral*
   I. Problems related to substance use or conjoint mental health services will continue *and* no current suicidal/homicidal ideation or history of uncontrolled aggression dangerous to others in last 30 days

(*continued*)

FIGURE 1. (*continued*)

II. Problems manageable at Level 2, or greater structure for assessment and mental health services is needed, or mild risk of endangering self/ others (includes fetus), increasing potential for uncontrolled aggressive behaviors

4. *Acceptance/resistance*
   I. Agreement to attend all scheduled activities, *or*, with or without admitting problems, monitoring and motivating strategies needed to identify treatment issues
   II. Extensive blaming, *or* more intensive services to be able to acknowledge alcohol and drug problems, *or* treatment failed at lower level

5. *Abstinence potential*
   I. Actively using and requires therapeutic intervention to achieve abstinence/sobriety, *or* has had some periods of abstinence, *or* unable to maintain abstinence or is at high risk to use and requires treatment to establish abstinence or minimize the risk of use
   II. High likelihood of use without intensive treatment by history, *or* lacks significant awareness of skills necessary to abstain and difficulty postponing immediate gratification despite Level 1 care, *or* inability to interrupt impulsive or high-risk behaviors that would threaten abstinence

6. *Recovery environment*
   I. Supportive environment exists *or* potential to develop adequate system exists
   II. Continued home/school exposure makes abstinence unlikely *or* significant proportion of peer group or leisure activities are drug involved

7. *Family functioning*
   I. Can maintain rules/expectations with minimal assistance *and* will abstain from problematic use and will participate in treatment process *and* transportation available
   II. Inconsistent ability to maintain rules *or* supportive but current conflicts interfere with client's treatment and need intervention to sustain a positive recovery environment *or* own use of chemicals problematic; they show an intermittent ability to abstain, yet will participate in treatment process

Finally, the provider should be comfortable making *multiple diagnoses*. Research has demonstrated that many psychiatric clients will have more than one diagnosis and addictions to several substances are common (Regier et al., 1990; Wolf et al., 1988). Women with preexisting posttraumatic stress disorder appear to be at an increased risk for both major depression and an alcohol use disorder (Breslau, Davis, Peterson, & Schultz, 1997). Not only is panic disorder often chronic, but also 25% of those with this disorder appear to go on to develop a major depression (Lydiard, Brawman-Mintzer, & Ballenger, 1996).

The convention is to list first the condition responsible for the evaluation or admission to clinical care. Do not let this convention, however, sway you from invoking the coexisting disorders model wherever applicable.

THE MENTAL STATUS EXAM

The mental status exam is a systematic procedure for making observations of intrapersonal dysfunction useful for establishing the psychiatric disorder of a dual diagnosis client. Although it is no substitute for a good history, the mental status exam helps to ensure a comprehensive evaluation of the client's feelings, thinking, and behavior. The exam also provides a means for bolstering assessment conclusions with specific observations that might suggest the need for further dual diagnosis evaluation and for communicating with other professionals. Chapters 6 and 7 list specific signs and symptoms associated with key Axis I diagnoses (see the tables in those two chapters).

The mental status exam covers the following areas:

1. *Appearance and behavior.* Look for poor or fastidious grooming, bizarre or deviant clothing, unusual or bizarre postures and mannerisms, facial expressions suggesting strong or unusual feelings.
2. *Attitude toward interview.* Look for suspicion, hostility, ingratiation, dependence, minimizing.
3. *Psychomotor activity.* Look for restlessness and agitation or for retardation, that is, general slowing of movement or speech.
4. *Affect and mood.* Look for flat, blunted affect with minimal display of emotion; lability, or rapid shifts of feelings; or inappropriate affect, where feelings seem incongruent with the content of the conversation or the situation. Look for excessively sad, euphoric, anxious, or angry affects.
5. *Speech and thought.* Look for rambling, loose, illogical, unconnected, or pressured speech. Look for bizarre content or suicidal and homicidal thoughts.
6. *Perceptual disturbances and hallucinations.* Look for responses to nonexistent sounds, sights, persons, and so forth.
7. *Orientation.* Ask and check for ability to state time (day, week, month, year), place (location of interview, name of city, county, etc.), person (self and interviewer), and situation with accuracy.
8. *Attention, concentration, and memory.* Check for ability to count backward by 7's from 100, to correctly repeat random strings of up to five to six digits forward and up to four to five backward (have these written out beforehand) or to spell the word "world"

backward; to repeat three unrelated objects or a new address and to recall these accurately after 5 minutes; to recall recent events that the interviewer can verify such as the current issues in the news or the waiting room's appearance; to recall remote events such as when certain historical events occurred or the names of the three presidents in office prior to the current president. Poor performance on these topics often suggests serious psychiatric difficulty. (Encourage depressed persons to try their best.)

9. *Intelligence.* Remembering to take education into account, look for high-level vocabulary or lack of same; look for concrete interpretations of proverbs after emphasizing to clients that you want them to state the meaning of the proverb in their own words. (e.g., Clinician: What does "Even monkeys fall out of trees" mean? Concrete response: "Monkeys can fall too." Abstract response: "Even experts make mistakes.")

10. *Reliability, insight, and judgment.* Estimate the client's cognitive functioning, motivation, and honesty; whether the client's behavior in various situations is likely to lead to negative outcomes; whether the client has some sense of present difficulties; and what some reasonable solutions might be.

Also useful is asking the client to copy a simple figure (such as a four-dimensional box or cross) to assess visual–motor deficits, something that is often missed in a verbal interview. Readers interested in additional reading about the mental status exam might find it helpful to read appropriate texts, such as the classic by Strub and Black (1985).

Although not part of the mental status exam, the "gut feeling" or intuition of the interviewer can also yield important diagnostic information. To the extent that the clinician successfully joins and paces with clients, the clinician's own state may somewhat mirror and match that of clients. Feeling weird, disjointed, and vaguely spacey in the interview can be a sign that clients are suffering from psychosis or dissociation. Feeling that the situation of the clients is overwhelming and hopeless can signal the presence of major depression. Feeling tense pressure to immediately relieve the suffering of clients is often common with those having anxiety disorders. Providers will get to know their own personal indicators of typical states with experience.

ASSESSING RISK OF HARM TO SELF OR OTHERS

A critical part of any psychiatric assessment is the evaluation of risk of harming oneself or others. The evaluator should always ask about suicidal (or self-harmful) and homicidal (or assaultive) thoughts and evaluate further if such thoughts are present. Asking will not put these thoughts into clients' heads. A matter-of-fact tone will facilitate inquiry into these matters. If such thoughts are present, the evaluator should inquire further about (1) the frequency and intensity of the thoughts, (2) whether clients have a specific plan and access to the means to carry the plan out, and (3) whether clients have a history of such behavior. Asking clients to rate themselves on whether they think their likelihood of acting on their thoughts is low, medium or high yields helpful information about the clients' own sense of self-control. Also helpful is asking clients what has prevented them from acting on their thoughts. A standard answer is what this would do to family and friends. This gives the clinician a possible strategic direction for intervention.

There are several predictors of risk (Bongar, 1991). The best predictor of risk is a previous history of behavior harmful to self or others. A specific plan and access to means is also a risk indicator, as is behavior consistent with taking action on their plans (e.g., giving away a valued pet). Degree of hopelessness is a predictor of suicide. Acute agitation, turmoil, or panic is a risk factor, as are command hallucinations (hallucinated orders to perform the harmful act). Social isolation increases risk. Recent losses or setbacks such as being fired or a spouse threatening a divorce are a risk factor. Another important indicator of risk is a recent psychiatric hospitalization. The risk further escalates significantly if a psychiatric condition or alcohol/drug intoxication (current or in the future) impairs the client's judgment and impulse control.

Antiharm contracts and perhaps increased outpatient contact are options for managing a low-risk client. The medium-risk client needs this, plus such measures as the certified removal of weapons or other means of violence from his/her possession and a 24-hour watch by family and friends. The high-risk client needs inpatient hospitalization or, if the situation is urgent, police involvement. Remember that the courts have decided that the duty to protect and warn other individuals when specific credible threats are made against them overrides clients' rights of confidentiality. Readers should check their own state laws and inquire with their state professional organization regarding this issue.

Consultation with a colleague or supervisor is often very useful in dealing with clients at risk for legal and professional reasons, not to mention personal ones. The colleague can help you think through the situation in a clearer fashion, support you emotionally, and serve as a witness. Documentation is also very important in order to communicate the situation to other professionals and, in the case of a lawsuit, support your side. You don't need to predict things perfectly; this is impossible. You do need to systematically assess the situation and intervene as indicated and document this.

A final word about whether clients are serious or merely "playing games" when they make threats. Our own personal policy is to treat all threats as serious. Guessing clients' "true" motivation is often not easy, and, besides, even game players accidentally kill themselves or others, misjudging the distance of those rocks underneath the bridge or mistakenly thinking that the safety lock on the gun pointed at the cheating spouse is on.

ISSUES IN ACHIEVING THE DIFFERENTIAL DIAGNOSIS WITH DUALLY DISORDERED CLIENTS

Making a differential diagnosis of the dually diagnosed client requires respect for the special issues surrounding the assessment of substance abuse and coexisting disorders as well as the investment of greater than usual time and energy.

We first need to consider base-rate issues. The Epidemiologic Catchment Area (ECA) Study found an overall lifetime prevalence rate for all disorders of 33% and that anxiety disorders were most common in the American population, with a lifetime prevalence of 15%, followed by substance use disorders at 17%, affective disorders at 8%, antisocial personality at 3%, cognitive impairment at 2%, and schizophrenic spectrum disorders at 2% (Regier, Farmer, Rae, Locke, et al., 1990). The same study found overall lifetime prevalence rates of any mental disorder in psychiatric hospitals as 82%, in prisons as 82% and in nursing homes as 66%, and substance use disorder rates of 34%, 72%, and 14%, respectively, in psychiatric hospitals, prisons, and nursing homes. Forty-seven percent of those suffering from schizophrenia met criteria for a substance use disorder, compared to 84% of those with antisocial personality disorder, 36% for panic disorders, 33% for obsessive–compulsive disorders, 13% for phobias, 60% for bipolar disorders, and approximately 30% for unipolar depression (the study did not, unfortunately, assess posttraumatic stress disorder). Almost 20% of those seen for treatment in mental health settings had a 6-month prevalence rate of substance use disorder, and 55% of those seen in chemical dependence treatment settings for an alcohol use disorder and 64% of those with a drug use disorder (other than alcohol) had a 6-month prevalence rate of comorbid mental health disorders.

The National Comorbidity Study, another recent epidemiological research project focusing on alcohol use disorders, found lifetime and 12-month prevalences of alcohol use disorders in the general population to be 9% and 3% respectively, with rates for men of alcohol abuse of 13% and 3% and for alcohol dependence of 20% and 7%, and rates for women of 6% and 2% for abuse and 8% and 2% for dependence (Kessler et al., 1997). Prior mental health disorders were more powerful predictors of subsequent alcohol dependence than alcohol abuse, and the majority of prior disorders were stronger predictors for women than men. Anxiety and affective disorders constituted the largest proportion of lifetime co-occurring cases among women, while substance use disorders, conduct disorder, and antisocial personality account for the majority of co-occurence among men. Of note is that, in this study, of those who had a lifetime diagnosis of alcohol abuse, 3% of men and 11% of women had a lifetime prevalence rate of posttraumatic stress disorder, as did 10% of men and 26% of women with a lifetime alcohol dependence diagnosis.

A review of the literature on diagnoses statistically associated with addiction problems identified the following (Bukstein, 1995): (1) conduct disorder in adolescents and antisocial personality disorder in adults; (2) attention deficit disorder; (3) major depression; (4) bipolar disorder; (5) anxiety disorder; (6) bulimia nervosa; (7) schizophrenia; and (8) borderline personality disorder.

The implications of these data are straightforward: dual disorders are extremely common. Evaluators in *chemical dependency treatment settings* must be prepared to assess for *probable* coexisting psychiatric disorders. Evaluators in *mental health settings* must be prepared to *rule out* a substance use disorder and in *settings treating chronically mentally ill* to also regard substance use disorders as *probable diagnoses*. The *index of suspicion* for active substance use disorders *goes up* for males compared to females, for younger clients, for males with a history of antisocial behavior, and for women with a history of anxiety and/or depression. And evaluators *need to take special care* when faced with a presentation of *the psychiatric disorders listed above* to evaluate for substance use disorders.

Another key point to keep in mind is that persons abusing or dependent on chemicals can evidence symptoms that mimic a host of psychiatric disorders. This can occur not only during acute intoxication from stimulants, hallucinogens, and other substances but also during withdrawal from alcohol and other substances. Substance-induced psychiatric syndromes can even affect substance abusers for periods of time past any obvious period of withdrawal. Sustained use of amphetamines can induce psychotic states, and withdrawal from amphetamines and cocaine can result in symptoms of an agitated depression. The hallucinogens can produce mood and psychotic or delusional disorders with varying courses. Cannabis use can trigger panic attacks and, with chronic use, a listless, amotivated status similar to dysthmia. Protracted withdrawal states that include mood, sleep, and cognitive disturbances can continue for months and even years, with the benzodiazepines especially notable for this (Ashton, 1995). Individuals abusing alcohol, opiates, sedative–hypnotics, and certain of the inhalants often show neuropsychological impairments and a variety of organic mental disorders including dementia (Geller, 1998). Even moderate levels of alcohol can substantially increase symptoms of anxiety and depression (Castenada et al., 1996). Levels of anxiety and depression high enough to qualify for a mental health diagnosis are very common among alcoholics, although more often than not these symptoms decrease with persistent abstinence (Kranzler, 1996; Brown et al., 1995).

Yet, these same studies show that, in the majority of cases, the concurrent psychiatric symptoms disappear with abstinence and time. Evaluators need to keep in mind that the "psychiatric" symptoms of their substance abusing clients may be attributable only to the chemical use and its consequences. An evaluator relying solely on reports and observations of signs of a psychiatric disorder when the individual has been abusing substances can overdiagnose a coexisting psychiatric disorder. Assessing for chemical use through client and collateral reports as well as biological assays (as described in Chapter 4) will assist in this process, as will using the diagnostic principles outlined in the next chapter.

At the same time, evaluators must still be prepared to make functional diagnoses of such problems as psychosis and suicidal ideation even if "only" due to substances and to make a plan for managing these problems. Evaluators must also be prepared to differentially diagnose any substance-induced psychiatric disorders. Simply assuming that treating the substance use disorder is sufficient is an unhelpful treatment bias. For example, one study found that clients with substance-induced psychiatric disorders had higher rates of rehospitalization and more substance-related impairment than dually diagnosed clients with "independent" psychiatric disorders—possibly because the first group did not receive mental health services but only drug and alcohol services (Dixon, McNary, & Lehman, 1997).

DIAGNOSTIC PRINCIPLES

How do we go about establishing that the client may have a psychiatric diagnosis in addition to a chemical dependency problem? In many cases a well-documented history or a clear-cut client presentation leaves no doubt regarding a coexisting psychiatric disorder. And despite the difficulties outlined above, even early research done in the area demonstrated that reliably assessing coexisting psychiatric disorders is quite possible (e.g., Penick, Powell, LIskow, Jackson, & Nickel, 1984). In our experience we have found seven decision rules (four major ones and three sudsidiary ones) useful in thinking through the data gleaned from clients' presentations and histories when the picture is less clear.

The first major rule is straightforward in principle: if the history indicates that the psychiatric difficulties began prior to the problematic chemical involvement (defined as heavy use and/or negative consequences), then consider the client to be dually disordered. While the coexisting disorders model is better for treatment purposes, this sort of primary–secondary distinction of the presenting problem can be useful for differential diagnosis and because the primary diagnosis seems to best predict the client's subsequent course (Tsuang, Cowley, Ries, Dunner, & Roy-Bryne, 1995; Schuckit, 1994). Using a collateral contact may help to get an accurate history, and emphasizing not individual symptoms but the age at which the individual met all criteria for a disorder may help to achieve a more accurate diagnosis (Schuckit, 1994).

The second major rule is that the symptoms and problems that clients present are qualitatively different from those usually seen with only problematic chemical involvement. These differences can include the intensity, frequency, or pattern of problems. Compared to individuals with drug-induced psychosis (Christie et al., 1988), persons with both schizophrenia and substance abuse/dependency are likely to show more classical signs of schizophrenia (e.g., poor insight, disorganized thoughts, and flat, blunted, or inappropriate affect), fewer signs of an organic mental disorder (e.g., disorientation, confusion, memory deficits, visual/tactile hallucinations); and longer duration of the psychosis prior to treatment contact (6 months). Compared to male alcoholics (Hesselbrock, Meyer, & Keener, 1985), persons with both substance abuse and antisocial personality demonstrated an earlier onset of both social difficulties and use of chemicals, a pattern of intense polysubstance abuse with rapid progression, and more legal system involvement. In one study, alcoholics with independent major depressive disorder were more likely to be married, European American, and female and to have had experience with fewer drugs, less treatment for alcoholism, to have attempted suicide, and to have a close relative with a major mood disorder (Schuckit, Tipp, Bergman, et al., 1997). In another study, alcoholics with comorbid major depression had higher suicidality (Cornelius et al., 1995).

The third principle is in some ways the best and in some ways the most controversial, namely, if the psychiatric problems continue during a chemical-free interval of 4 weeks after detox, then consider a second diagnosis. The period of abstinence can be determined either by information about clients' histories or during a period of ongoing treatment and observation. A period of abstinence of sufficient length usually removes the chemical involvement as a confounding factor. A few patients with protracted withdrawal symptoms do show chronic symptoms apparently caused by just the chemical use, but generally this rule works well.

The controversial aspect involves the length of time that the client must be abstinent to be certain that the client was not still toxic and under the influence. We have chosen the 4-week criterion for a number of reasons. First, our medical lab consultants tell us that even the psychoactive ingredient of THC in marijuana, notorious for staying in the body for several weeks because of its affinity for storage in fat tissues, is no longer detectable in the urine of most chronic daily pot smokers after 30 days. Second, a number of neurological indices return to normal after 30 days of abstinence (Geller, 1998; Volkow et al., 1994). Third, research data and clinical experience indicate that many of the "psychiatric" symptoms caused by the chemical abuse will subside during this time period (Kranzler, 1996; Brown et al., 1995).

The fourth decision rule is to use the formal DSM-IV diagnostic criteria to diagnose the psychiatric disorder. Deciding whether the client suffers from an independent major depression presents a good example. Many individuals with substance use disorders complain of "small d" depression, that is, of being down, "blue," and so forth. However, these individuals will not meet the diagnostic criteria for labeling the condition a major depression. Using the DSM-IV criteria appears to improve diagnostic accuracy (Schuckit, Tipp, Bergman, et al., 1997).

We never use alone the three subsidiary rules that follow to establish the second diagnosis. But we do use them to confirm and support a "yes" decision based on the four major rules. We also use these subsidiary rules as tiebreakers when the major rules produce a "maybe." The first subsidiary rule is that the client has a family history that supports the psychiatric diagnosis under consideration. There is a genetic component to such diagnoses as schizophrenia, bipolar disorder, some anxiety and depressive disorders, and—at least for depression and alcoholism—the independent genetic transmission of the two disorders (Schuckit, 1994). The second subsidiary rule is that the client has a history of multiple treatment failures in standard chemical dependency or mental health treatment programs. We base this rule on our clinical experience that these clients have difficulty in staying in treatment and in not relapsing. Typical failures may include leaving before completion of treatment, substantial noncompliance with program rules, and relapses during or after treatment. Rather than view these difficulties as a lack of motivation for recovery, we consider the possibility of a second diagnosis. The third subsidiary rule is the person's response to a trial of (nonaddictive) neuroleptic medication. Especially when psychological testing done several weeks after detox indicates a possible psychiatric disorder and the "psychiatric" symptoms continue, a positive patient response to a medication that treats a disorder gives support to the person's having that disorder.

Making psychiatric diagnoses is a slippery art, especially with potentially dually disordered patients. Getting a good history can be difficult. The most common coexisting anxiety disorders are very difficult to distinguish from similar symptoms caused by chemical usage (Kranzler, 1996). Differences among symptoms caused solely by chemical use and not a psychiatric disorder are more difficult to assess in an outpatient environment than in an inpatient setting (Tsuang et al., 1995). Nonetheless, these decision rules can guide clinicians into more accurate diagnoses.

TREATMENT DECISIONS

As noted in the preceding section, sometimes the functional or working diagnosis determines treatment disposition in acute or crisis situations while the true "primary" diagnosis is left undefined for the time being. The client experiencing an acute psychosis or intense suicidal or homicidal ideation—even if it has been caused only by chemical use—will require psychiatric management. However, establishing whether or not a coexisting psychiatric disorder exists has important long-term consequences. It is one thing to stabilize the chemically induced "psychiatric" problem and then refer the patient to a chemical dependency treatment program. It's another thing entirely to decide that the person will need both chemical dependency services and mental health services for the foreseeable future.

In some cases the person may have an established but stable psychiatric disorder. Many people suffering from bipolar disease, for example, are well controlled on medication and can benefit from a standard chemical dependency program. Many people also have "mild" cases of a disorder and can tolerate and benefit from typical programs treating the substance abuse or dependency disorder. Our general preference is to refer to a chemical dependency program whenever possible. The person will receive more focused attention to his/her currently acute chemical use problem, and there will be a reduced risk of the program focusing only on the mental health problem. These programs are also less expensive and involve fewer restrictions on the client. However, certain situations demand dual diagnosis treatment containing both chemical dependency and mental health treatment components.

Ries and Miller (1993) have proposed a typology of dually diagnosed clients to assist in treatment planning. They first view treatment as having acute, subacute, and long-term phases, with the corresponding care systems of emergency rooms/acute inpatient units, inpatient/intensive outpatient, and outpatient settings. They define four groups of clients with dual disorders and associated treatment needs. Type I clients have high psychiatric severity and high substance severity. They require emergency room and acute psychiatric inpatient care in the acute and subacute phases and integrated treatment in the long-term phase. Type II clients have high psychiatric severity and low substance severity. These clients can benefit from an integrated program with supplementary chemical dependency intervention. Type III clients have low psychiatric severity and high substance severity. These clients, once psychiatrically stable, can go to inpatient or intensive outpatient chemical dependency treatment with psychiatric consultation available if the psychiatric disorder remains unresolved. Type IV clients have low psychiatric severity and low substance severity and can benefit from outpatient counseling that is preferably integrated.

The American Society of Addiction Medicine (ASAM; 1996) criteria are a detailed set of admission and continuing stay and discharge criteria that are widely used in the chemical dependency treatment field and by third-party payors (American Society of Addiction Medicine, 1996). The criteria provide for five levels of care: Level 0.5, early intervention; Level I, outpatient; Level II, intensive outpatient/partial hospital; Level III, residential; and Level IV, medically managed intensive inpatient. The criteria ask the evaluator to make judgments on six independent dimensions: acute intoxication/withdrawal potential; biological conditions/complications; emotional/behavioral conditions; treatment acceptance/resistance; relapse/continue use potential, and recovery/living environment. For adolescents, there is a seventh dimension involving the family's ability to support treatment. The Client Intake Tool (Figure 1), provides some of the specific language of the criteria for Level I and Level II outpatient treatment. The criteria for Level III acknowledge directly the impact of any psychiatric disorder, and the other criteria can indirectly take the psychiatric disorder into account. Some professionals believe that the ASAM criteria can accommodate the client with dual disorders (e.g., Molly, 1992). Our own experience is that the system tends to minimize the role of the psychiatric disorder and of the acute psychiatric inpatient treatment program. Nonetheless, the ASAM criteria are the standard in the field and the most sophisticated set of treatment guidelines provided to date, and we use them for our own clients, even addressing these dimensions when we treat mental-health-only clients.

CHAPTER 6

The Psychotic and Cognitive Disorders

There are those too who suffer from grave emotional
and mental disorders.
They too are able to recover if they have the capacity
for honesty.
> —From "How It Works" (*Big Book* of
> Alcoholics Anonymous)

This chapter focuses on treating psychotic disorders or cognitive disorders
with coexisting chemical dependency. For each diagnosis we discuss the
typical presenting symptoms and problems that individuals with these
diagnoses evidence. All diagnostic criteria and most of the information
on prognosis are from DSM-IV except where there are separate citations
(see American Psychiatric Association, 1994). For each set of diagnoses
we review general mental health treatment strategies. We then devote
extensive portions of our discussion to the counseling approach that, in
our experience, is useful in helping these clients achieve dual recovery
from both chemical dependency and the psychiatric disorder. We focus
especially on the early stages of recovery. We have included examples of
stepwork for each set of diagnoses in Appendix 1.

CLIENTS WITH A SCHIZOPHRENIC OR OTHER PSYCHOTIC DISORDER

Diagnostic Features

A great challenge for the treatment professional is the person who suffers from schizophrenia and who also suffers from a substance use disorder. Severe symptoms, multiple needs, limited resources, and organizational barriers contribute to this challenge.

The cardinal features of schizophrenia include substantial impairment of clients' thought processes as well as the bizarre content of their thought. DSM-IV states that two or more of the following symptoms must be present during a significant portion of time during a 1-month period to diagnose schizophrenia: delusions; hallucinations; disorganized speech; grossly disorganized or catatonic behavior; and "negative symptoms." Catatonic is a catchall term for a variety of unusual symptoms involving unusual movements and can include immobility, excessive and agitated movements, being mute, posturing, stereotyped movements and parroting of other people's words or mirroring their behavior. Positive symptoms are a problem because of what *is* there, such as hallucinations and delusions. Negative symptoms are problems because of what *is not* there. Negative symptoms include alogia, or brief, concrete replies to questions and little spontaneous speech (poverty of speech) and speech that conveys little information because it is vague, repetitive, overly abstract, or stereotyped (poverty of content). Other negative symptoms include affective flattening, or very muted emotional expressiveness, and avolition, or inability to initiate and persist in goal-directed activities. Symptoms must be present for a minimum of 6 months to make the diagnosis of schizophrenia, and there must be a decline in psychosocial functioning.

The condition also tends to be chronic, with flareups in response to stress, failure to take medications, or chemical use. Onset is typically in late adolescence or early adulthood. Complete remission is not common, and many persons with this devastating illness deteriorate over time. Negative symptoms in particular tend to be chronic and increase with time (McGlashan & Fenton, 1992). Ten percent of persons suffering from this disorder will commit suicide. The prognosis for women is better than for men. Subtypes of schizophrenia (determined by the most prominent feature of the presenting clinical picture) include paranoid, disorganized, catatonic, undifferentiated (does not meet any of the foregoing descriptions) and residual (negative symptoms only) types. Table 2 lists other significant features of the schizophrenic disorder.

Other psychotic disorders include (1) schizophreniform disorder, where the schizophrenic symptoms have lasted less than 6 months and where there is not necessarily a decline in functioning; (2) schizoaffective disorder, where mood and active-phase symptoms of schizophrenia occur concurrently after 2 weeks of delusions or hallucinations without prominent mood symptoms; (3) brief psychotic disorder, which lasts more than 1 day but remits by 1 month; (4) delusional disorder, with delusions only; and (5) psychotic conditions that are substance-induced or due to a medical condition.

TABLE 2. Schizophrenia

Feelings	Thinking	Behavior	Interpersonal relations and role functioning
Generally inappropriate or muted Can be very depressed or angry or anxious	Confusion Difficulty concentrating Concrete and unable to generalize information Bizarre content, delusions Hallucinations Somatic preoccupation Greater impairment in auditory modalities	Disorganized Decreased responsiveness to others Eccentric Poor grooming/routine	Withdrawn and isolated Poor role functioning May be able to do low-pressure jobs requiring little contact with public

A classic dilemma for achieving a differential diagnosis is the client with a presentation and course that suggest schizophrenia (including both negative and positive symptoms) following severe polysubstance abuse, especially amphetamines or other stimulants. Did the stimulant use create the disorder or merely trigger a latent vulnerability? Explanations of this phenomenon usually invoke the well-documented research finding of neurological "sensitization," when less and less of a drug is needed to provoke a response (the opposite of tolerance) and "cross-sensitization," when responses to other drugs and stressors in general are exaggerated (Flaum & Schultz, 1996). Symptoms associated with amphetamine use can develop several months after cessation of use and take up to five or more years to resolve. The clinician's best strategy at this point is to adopt a "time will tell" stance and base the treatment plan on the functional needs and problems of the client. These individuals are often more amenable to treatment than many persons with schizophrenia, because they bring personal strengths and skills to the treatment (including ease in relating to other people) not always found in those suffering from schizophrenia. They also tend to have an appreciation of the losses caused by their chemical use, which makes denial busting somewhat easier (but also makes the risk of suicide higher).

Key Treatment Issues

There are three key issues in managing the person with schizophrenia and other serious psychotic disorders (e.g., Ayuso-Gutierrez & del Rio Vega, 1997; Haywood et al., 1995). The first is medication compliance. Antipsychotic medications have the primary and necessary role in the treatment of these disorders (Breslin, 1992). Persons suffering from these disorders must take medication regularly to control their psychotic symptoms. Trade names of some commonly used antipsychotic medications used in the past include Haldol, Navane, Prolixin, Stelazine, Thorazine, Loxitane, and Trilafon. Other medications have recently become available that appear to be more effective than the older ones in that they address not only the positive but also the negative symptoms of the schizophrenic-type conditions (Meltzer, 1993). And they do so with fewer side effects. Resperdal (resperidone) is one example of such a medication (Cardone, 1995). Other new antipsychotic medications of this sort are Zyprexa (olanzapine) and Seroquel (quetiapine). Clozaril(clozapine) is a medication that is often helpful for persons who are neuroleptic-resistant or -intolerant but requires careful, expensive monitoring because of the risk of agranulocytosis (Rosenheck et al., 1999; Buchanan, Breier, Kirkpatrick, Ball, & Carpenter, 1998). However, persons suffering from schizophrenia and similar disorders often stop taking their medications. This is a prime contributor to relapse (e.g. Robinson et al., 1999; Reynolds et al., 1999). Sometimes the side effects of the medication are uncomfortable. Individuals with schizophrenia can also be suspicious of the medication or remain unconvinced that they are ill and require the medication. Or sometimes the person becomes so disorganized that nothing gets done in a routine fashion.

The second issue is the disabilities that are associated with schizophrenia and similar disorders and that lead to marked deficits in role performance. Persons with these kinds of illnesses have trouble with their concentration and short-term memory, have difficulty thinking abstractly and translating information and a plan into behavior, and often do not experience such positive emotions as the "joy of achievement." Schizophrenia is associated with generalized cognitive deficits. The negative symptoms, in particular, are associated with impaired learning (MacPherson, Jerrom, & Hughes, 1996; Mueser, Bellack, & Blanchard, 1992). Individuals with these kinds of disorders often have difficulty performing activities of daily living, including even such basic ones as eating and grooming. These persons can find that attending scheduled events such as clinic appointments, job interviews, and so forth are quite beyond them. They are very vulnerable to even normal stress and have problems using and even tolerating social support even when taking medication (Butzlaff & Hooley,

1998; Buchanan, 1995; Norman & Malla, 1993). The results of all this can include downward "drift" into marginal jobs or unemployment, estrangement from families and friends, homelessness, and serious medical problems.

The third issue is the need for abstinence from alcohol and drugs and treatment for this as indicated. As we have seen in Chapter 5, almost half of those with this disorder have in their lifetime experienced a substance use disorder, with estimates of recent or current use ranging from 20% to 40% (Regier et al., 1990; Mueser et al., 1992). Studies support demographic and environmental factors (especially availability) as accounting for the exact substances used among those suffering from schizophrenia, and the studies doe not support self-medication for selected symptoms (e.g., el-Guebaly & Hodgins, 1992; Mueser et al., 1992). Those with comorbid substance use disorders, in fact, may have a history of higher premorbid functioning that effectively increased their exposure to drug-using situations (Arndt, Tyrrell, Flaum, & Andreasen, 1992).

Substance use disorders interact with schizophrenic and other disorders to exacerbate symptoms, multiply problems, and complicate treatment. Persons suffering from schizophrenia who also abuse substances, for example, have higher rates of hallucinations, and the perceptual distortions are more treatment refractory (Brunnette, Mueser, Xie, & Drake, 1997; Sokolski et al., 1994). Even moderate drinking appears to be unsafe for this population (Drake & Wallach, 1993). These clients have higher utilization rates of hospital and jail services and higher rates of homelessness, although not necessarily because of any direct exacerbation of symptoms (Haywood et al., 1995; Bartels et al., 1993; Caton, Wyatt, Felix, Grunber, & Dominguez, 1993). These clients have lower rates of medication compliance and contact with outpatient resources (Owen, Fischer, Booth, & Cuffel, 1996). Treatment that integrates mental health and chemical dependency services has better outcomes with this population (e.g., Drake, Yovetich, Bebout, Harris, & McHugo, 1997).

General Treatment Strategies and Tactics

When counseling clients with both a psychotic and a substance use disorder, remember that you are dealing with brain diseases that impair thinking both in the short term and often in the long term. And remember that medication and abstinence are necessary to control the symptoms of schizophrenia and its associated problems. Until the medication is at adequate levels, use techniques such as a time-out in the person's room or contacts that are brief to keep social stimulation low. Even with adequate medication, the person suffering from schizophrenia can quickly disorganize in response to just moderate stress (Norman & Malla,

1993). One well-researched source of stress materializes whenever these other persons around the client show intense affect and demand high levels of performance that the person with schizophrenia cannot possibly deliver (Liberman & Corrigan, 1993). Use a passive, friendly, low-key approach, minimizing high levels of confrontation, challenge, and criticism. Give feedback in a matter-of-fact style. Half-hour appointments and 45-minute groups often work best. Keep treatment goals modest and take a long-term perspective. Be prepared to go very slowly with the introduction of diagnostic labels, especially with clients suffering from paranoia. Phrasing issues as "problems with anxiety" instead of psychosis and describing consequences as "ending up in hospitals after smoking pot and taking speed" rather than addiction are a good way to begin to work on increasing your client's insight.

Persons with schizophrenia typically have trouble learning new information, especially when presented in auditory modalities, and translating this into new behavior. Use lots of visual aids and throw away step study audiotapes, as those require too much concentration for these clients. Keep material simple and concrete. Do not assume that clients can perform even the basics, and be comprehensive. Consistent with this, one study found that medication compliance was not improved with simple instruction but did increase with a comprehensive, step-by-step orientation to each individual step in the chain of "taking your medications," including such things as the use of pill containers, calendars for appointments, and so forth (Cramer & Rosenheck, 1999; Azrin & Teichner, 1998). Think repetition, repetition, repetition. Clients with these disorders will need repeated exposure to basic facts and information as well as repeated opportunities to practice new skills. Repetition is also the basis for these clients to understand the connection between substance use and negative consequences. Help the client apply new material to each specific situation. Use modeling to demonstrate the behavior, and have the client role-play the behavior. Above all, keep it simple.

Also think structure, structure, structure. Written prompts such as checklists for activities of daily living and hour-by-hour time schedules are useful. Groups that have a topical focus and use classroom methods are more likely to be helpful than process groups (Kahn & Kahn, 1992). Even with these aids, persons suffering from schizophrenia will most definitely benefit from supervision by a case manager who can remind, prompt, and assist them. Assertive outreach and intensive case management are usually necessary to keep these clients and others suffering from chronic mental illness engaged and on track (Gorey et al., 1998; Drake & Noordsy, 1994). Many people with schizophrenia will require on-the-spot supervision in a residential home placement or day-treatment program. Where resources and the structure are available, token economies (points, chips, etc., earned for behavior and then exchanged for rewards) have proven helpful and have even been blended with 12-step approaches (Liberman & Kopelowicz, 1995; Fanco, 1995).

Several tricky dynamics often arise in counseling clients with schizophrenia. Paranoia provides a notable example. Early in treatment we "join" (express empathy) with the profound fear of these clients and then shift the emphasis to the need to take medication for the overwhelming anxiety. We avoid direct challenges to any delusions. Later on, we adopt an intellectual "let's examine all the relevant hypotheses and, in fact, let's agree to disagree" attitude toward delusions. Later still, we label delusions as symptoms and agree that, while the feelings of persecution are a fact, the persecution itself is not a fact. The goal here is to very, very gradually make the delusions seem as unreal, while acknowledging the fearful reality of them for clients as part of their illness.

Many clients suffering from schizophrenia develop a profound demoralization as they experience the enormous impact this illness has on their lives, lives that are (in many cases) supposed to be entering the full, glorious bloom of the twenties. Expressing admiration for their strength in coping, asking clients what keeps them going and amplifying on this, and locating alternative sources of satisfaction and meaning are strategies for this demoralization. Moreover, rates of comorbid major depression and suicidal ideation are high among those suffering from schizophrenia (Wassink, Flaum, Nopoulos, & Andreasen, 1999). Assessing, monitoring, and treating these disorders and problems are important tasks.

Denial of either or both illnesses can be handled with education and rational discussion, as well as presentation of the facts of the assessment, carefully titrated to the client's functional level. Education regarding the disease of schizophrenia and of substance dependence and ultimately meeting others with both these illnesses can help to combat the stigma that still remains around these disorders. Professionals will also need their own sources of support as they face the toll of these illnesses day in and day out.

When stable, the person suffering from schizophrenia benefits from socialization activities. This helps to keep him/her oriented and involved with others and provides support for coping with his/her illness. Don't be surprised, however, at the almost allergic reaction these clients have to socialization activities. Other human beings are a source of great rewards but also of great stress. A low-key, drop-in format can help engage clients unwilling or unable to engage in anything more intensive. Many persons with less severe schizophrenia can also benefit from skills training and practice in such areas as taking the bus, balancing a checkbook, and preparing meals. Other useful training focuses on simple social skills such as carrying on a conversation and perhaps even on-job training for simple jobs that have a consistent routine and are not overly stressful.

Families of dually diagnosis persons with schizophrenia benefit from education about both illnesses, the schizophrenia and the chemical abuse. Intervention with the family also decreases the relapse rates of clients and improved outcomes above and beyond that of medication (Baucom, Shoham, Mueser, Daiuto, & Stickle, 1998; Schooler, 1995). Families also require help in setting realistic expectations for what the person suffering from schizophrenia and a substance use disorder can do. Families must walk the fine line between making unrealistic demands and enabling the family member by rescuing him/her from the failure to stay abstinent and take his/her medications. Discussions with family members about the hazards of chemical use can help challenge such statements as a family member's saying, "What's wrong with a little beer and pot? He has so little else in his life." Contingency plans around scenarios such as "What do I do when my son shows up drunk and psychotic on my doorstep?" are necessary. Families also benefit from referral to support groups such as the National Alliance for the Mentally Ill and Alanon (see p. 186, in Chapter 10). The burden, both financial and emotional, on families is often enormous, and the question of "Who cares for the caretakers?" is a pertinent one (Clark, 1994).

In our experience inpatient hospitalization is usually necessary to stabilize acute schizophrenia and begin recovery. Managing acute psychosis and maintaining early abstinence are often impossible on an outpatient basis. A comprehensive outpatient continuing care program following inpatient care is also imperative for long-term success. Some individuals with psychotic symptoms and a substance use will respond quickly to just education about their dual illnesses with medication compliance and abstinence, but in our experience this is distressingly uncommon. Additional measures are often necessary. External strategies for managing the situation involve the administration of medications by other persons (such as a residential home manager) or even shots of long-lasting injectable medication. Some living arrangements may make it possible to try to restrict access to chemicals, but this is often not successful. Designating a third-party payee for social security disability benefits (where applicable) can often help to restrict access to chemicals through control of financial resources. Such measures as these can provide the sobriety and stability necessary for education and counseling tactics to take hold.

Substance Disorder Counseling

Doing a comprehensive chemical dependency assessment with someone who is psychotic can be a waste of time. Your best bet is to interview significant others (especially case managers) and ask whether the client uses any type of drug or alcohol. In our experience and that of others, rates of both alcohol and marijuana use are high, apparently because these are easily accessible (e.g., Cuffel, Heithoff, & Lawson, 1993). If there is any report of chemical use, even just alcohol or marijuana, the person may need dual diagnosis treatment, especially if the person does not remain abstinent after instructions to avoid chemicals. Any use of alcohol and drugs is contraindicated for the person with schizophrenia. Marijuana is a real problem. Our own clinical experience suggests that persons with schizophrenia who smoke marijuana, even when taking proper doses of medication, often experience a psychotic episode. When abusing alcohol schizophrenics tend to discontinue their medications, since the alcohol further disorganizes them and exacerbates the side effects of the medication.

Occasionally we have seen a few patients who abused their side-effect medication because of the buzz that anticholinergic agents such as Artane can deliver. Watch out for those clients who run out of their side-effect medication before their antipsychotic medication. They could be using (or selling) the anticholinergic medication. Using other medications for these side effects such as Sinemet avoids this problem or, perhaps better yet, switching clients to one of the newer medications is certainly another option. Some psychiatrists also prescribe a potentially addictive antianxiety agent such as Valium or Xanax to control agitation or any exacerbation of symptoms, often with good results (Carpenter, Buchanan, Kirkpatrick, & Breier, 1999). This should generally be avoided, however, when working with the dually diagnosed person with schizophrenia because of cross-tolerance, cross-dependence, and the highly addictive nature of benzodiazepines. These medications can also be associated with strong anxiety rebound effects when discontinued.

Persons with schizophrenia often have strong denial about the effects of alcohol and drugs on their lives, not unlike other drug and alcohol abusers. However, pounding on their denial through heavy confrontation is not appropriate. Strong confrontation will lead to further exacerbation of psychotic symptoms. Instead, the task of the recovery counselor is to slowly and painfully build into the client's world view that he/she is chemically dependent and cannot use drugs or alcohol at all, ever, under any circumstances. Explaining that chemical dependency is a disease helps give persons with schizophrenia a clear and concrete rationale why no use of chemicals is necessary, as they suffer from the disease of chemical dependency. If we can convince the person with schizophrenia that he/she is chemically dependent and that he/she needs to be abstinent, we are satisfied with our work. We do not expect him/her to complete the first five steps in the first 30 days of sobriety.

We have modified our stepwork for this client. Our Step 1 focuses on unmanageability. We are clear and concrete. We stay away from too much emphasis on powerlessness, as this can lead to further disorganization in the thinking of this population (see Appendix 1 for an example of stepwork for persons with schizophrenia). For clients with denial about their schizophrenic illness, we include the equivalent of Step 1 activities on symptoms of this illness.

We often ask clients suffering from schizophrenia to develop two sets of cue cards as part of their Step 1 work. We first educate them about the differences between needed medications (good drugs) and bad drugs (such as marijuana). We then assist them in writing out three reasons why they need to take their medications and three reasons why they cannot use drugs. Often these reasons are very basic, such as "I'll end up in hospitals like this" or "I'll lose my housing." Checking with the referral source or case manager will help generate valid, pertinent reasons. We ask the person with schizophrenia to write these reasons on the cue cards and then to carry these cards. Our staff frequently ask them to state three reasons for needing to take medications and to state three reasons why they should stop using chemicals. We refer them back to the cards until the clients can state the reasons with minimal prompting. Using pictures of negative consequences cut out from magazines (e.g., jail) helps the less verbal person.

Doing Steps 2 and 3 with persons with psychosis can be a challenge. Spending too much time on vague or rambling discussions of a Higher Power, the "Force," "God speaking to me now," and so forth is at best a waste of time and at worst can reinforce psychotic thinking. We approach these issues with a gentle touch, joining with the client around how important these issues are to him or her and then redirecting the client to more day-to-day practical matters and details. The latter might include identifying other specific persons or activities that might be helpful to the client and how, by letting go and letting others help, the client cannot be alone and without assistance in the attempt to stay sober and stable. Later in treatment, we help more stabilized clients to recognize the difference between a spiritual approach to life and a delusional religious preoccupation.

We encourage clients to attend chemical dependency groups on an inpatient basis as soon as they show evidence of stabilized thinking. Often 72 hours of adequate doses of neuroleptic medication will begin to make a difference in their thinking. They benefit from repeated exposure to material and the support for abstinence they will find in a well-functioning group. We sometimes wait longer on an outpatient basis.

The counselor must also establish a norm of tolerance for unusual behavior in the group (especially a mixed group of people with different diagnoses) but also be ready to set limits and keep stimulation levels low. The counselor will need to supplement group work with a great deal of individual attention, especially if the person with schizophrenia continues to have difficulty in participating in a group format. Supportive one-on-one counseling also appears to be helpful in and of itself as part of the treatment plan, as is problem-solving therapy with better-recovered patients (Tarrier et al., 1998; Gunderson et al., 1984; Goldberg, Schooler, Hogarty, & Roper, 1977).

The person with schizophrenia most often benefits from a sympathetic AA group or, if available, a dual recovery or double trouble group. The counselor should be familiar with AA groups that are more tolerant of medication use and unusual behavior. The counselor will also want to warn the person with schizophrenia that some individuals might question his/her use of medication and help him/her to develop and rehearse statements to rebut these comments. We suggest assisting the client in getting a supportive AA sponsor who can meet with the counselor and the patient to discuss the medication issue. We also give the client the pamphlet on medications and their role in recovery published by AA. In situations where appropriate groups are not available, professionals can ask for help from the institutional committee of the local AA organization in identifying a person in the program who might be willing to help start a group on site or can use a higher functioning client to do the same thing. Some sort of group support is important, and, whatever form it takes, providing clients with this backup is important.

Relapse Prevention

Clients with schizophrenia who had achieved symptom and residential stability appear to benefit from a relapse intervention called personal therapy by its originators (Hogarty et al., 1997). This intervention has three phases. Phase 1 involves supportive counseling, psychoeducation, problem solving, social skills practice, and medication management. Phase 2, often entered into only 18 months after discharge from the hospital, involves identifying individual indicators of negative affect and skills (such as relaxation techniques) to manage negative feelings, as well as continued social skills training. The third, advanced, phase involves social and vocational initiatives in the community, awareness of triggers for problems and other self-monitoring skills, and work on clients' social impact on others. Of note is the fact that those not living with families or in a stable living situation actually become worse with personal therapy, apparently because of the stress of dealing with basic issues of food, clothing, shelter, and so forth. These results support the outside-in strategy and need for long-term treatment of dually diagnosed clients, discussed in earlier chapters. While the research cited above on personal therapy did not focus specifically on dually diagnosed clients, certainly this paradigm could easily be expanded to include substance use. Our own experience is that isolation and boredom as well as lack of structure are key triggers for substance use that should be addressed in working with clients to develop "just in case" plans to forestall relapse. Our attitude toward relapse is one that views it as a failure in the treatment plan, not the person, and we join with clients in the search for a solution to the problem of the relapse. The relapse becomes a priority for work in the treatment sessions but not an opportunity for blaming and shaming of clients.

Do not expect miracles, but do not give up prematurely. Many persons with schizophrenia, especially with ongoing comprehensive support services, stay abstinent and stable. Some, however, take two steps forward and one step back, but they do slowly progress on the road to recovery.

CLIENTS WITH DEMENTIA AND OTHER COGNITIVE DISORDERS

Diagnostic Features

Formerly included under the rubric of organic mental disorders, the cognitive disorders refer primarily to delirium, dementia, and amnesic disorders. These disorders are associated with a significant deficit in cognition or memory that represents a change from previous functioning. The cause of the disorder is a general medical condition, a substance, or some combination of the two.

The diagnostic criteria for delirium include (1) a disturbance of consciousness with reduced ability to focus, sustain, or shift attention; (2) a change in cognition, such as memory deficit, disorientation, or language disturbance, or the development of a perceptual disturbance that is not better accounted for by an evolving dementia; (3) the development of the disturbance over a short period of time (usually hours to days), with a tendency to fluctuate during the course of the day; and (4) evidence that there is a medical cause. Delirium can be caused by an acute infection or by intoxication caused by recent use of psychoactive or other chemicals or withdrawal from such substances. Diagnostic criteria for dementia include memory impairment as well as at least one of the following symptoms of cognitive disturbance: (1) disturbances in understanding or producing ideas in language involving reading, writing, or speaking; (2) an inability to carry out motor activities and routines; (3) failure to recognize or identify objects despite intact sensory function; or (4) difficulties in planning, executing, or monitoring complex activities or in solving problems. The diagnostic criteria for an amnesic disorder includes impaired memory functions, leading to difficulty learning new information or being unable to recall previously learned information or past events.

We limit our discussion here to the mild to moderate and chronic dementias. Dementia is the prototypical cognitive disorder that raises issues of the need for dual diagnosis treatment. The essential features of dementia are memory difficulties and other cognitive impairments as well as profound personality deterioration. Table 3 presents the signs and symptoms of dementia in more detail. Delirium, acute withdrawal, severe intoxification, and severe dementia require medical and nursing management to ensure safety and health. Care providers will most likely need to deal with dually diagnosed persons experiencing the less transient disorders associated with prolonged chemical use or other etiological factors.

Key Treatment Issues

As we have discussed in the preceding chapter, some chemically abusing or dependent individuals can evidence a protracted withdrawal syndrome lasting not just weeks but months and even years. Anxiety, depression, cognitive difficulties, physiological symptoms such as sleep disturbance,

TABLE 3. Dementia

Feeling	Thinking	Behavior	Interpersonal relations and role functioning
Sometimes anxiety or depression	Short- and long-term memory impairment	Often poor impulse control, with actions that are potentially harmful	Often conflict with others
Sometimes apathy or indifference	Impaired abstract thinking and judgment	Often outbursts, tantrums, assaults	Impairment in work and social activities, poor coping with stressors
Sometimes lability and irritability	Impaired auditory–verbal and/or visual–motor abilities	Sometimes disorganized or perseverative behavior	In serious cases, impaired activities of daily living
	Impaired short- and long-term memory	Change or exaggeration in personality style	
	Sometimes paranoid thinking		
	Slower information processing		

irritability, emotional lability, and transient or chronic psychotic symptoms can characterize this syndrome (e.g., Kinney & West, 1996). Receptor imaging techniques, for example, have shown that there are persistent changes in dopamine receptors in cocaine addicts even in abstinence that can last for months and that are associated with a residual mood disorder (Volkow, Fowler, & Wolf, 1991, cited in O'Brien, 1996). Relapse back into drinking and using, then, may not be just a matter of denial but a consequence of ongoing neurophysiological impairment that clouds thinking, perturbs emotions, and disrupts coping behavior.

Well researched are the cognitive deficits observed even in abstinent alcoholics that can last for years, especially in older alcoholics (Fein, Bachman, Fisher, & Davenport, 1990). Females may be more susceptible to alcohol's effects on neuropsychological functioning (Nixon & Glenn, 1995). The more severe deficits are in the areas of visuospatial abilities, perceptual–motor integration, abstract reasoning, and new learning. Cocaine users, at least in the short term, also show impaired cognitive abilities (Beatty, Katzung, Moreland, & Nixon, 1995). The existence of a prolonged withdrawal syndrome associated with marijuana and characterized, among other things, by memory problems is controversial and the evidence mixed (Pope, Gruber, & Yurgelun-Todd, 1995). The research on inhalant users has also found evidence for cognitive damage as a group (Byrne, Kirby, Zibin, & Ensminger, 1991). Polysubstance use may be associated with the greatest persistence of at least cognitive difficulties (Selby & Azrin, 1998). Not only substance use but other factors could account for these deficits. These include accidents resulting in head trauma, poor nutrition, liver disease, and other medical complications, as well as genetic factors that might contribute either to the development of a generalized dementia or an amnesic syndrome (Goldman, 1990). Sons of alcoholics, for example, show distinct cognitive difficulties, including deficits in attention and concentration, on a variety of measures even before significant exposure to alcohol (Schuckit, 1989).

Cognitive deficits, not surprisingly, are a barrier to recovery. Lower levels of cognitive functioning in alcoholics are associated with lowered rates of completing treatment programs, less success in work environments after discharge, and reduced duration of clean and sober time after discharge (Goldman, 1990). Neurocognitive performance and depressive symptoms together appear to especially predict increased relapse behavior after discharge among alcoholics (Parsons, 1998). One study found that lower levels of verbal learning was associated with poorer drinking outcomes among alcoholics receiving relapse prevention training but not supportive therapy (Jaffe et al., 1996). This implies that a poor match between cognitive abilities and psychotherapy intervention might produce iatrogenic deterioration.

General Treatment Strategies and Tactics

Generally standard chemical dependency programs and staff have experience in dealing with clients who have substance use disorders and are experiencing very mild dementia. Adequate nutrition, reassurance and support, and, most especially, the passage of time with ongoing abstinence manages this adequately, with many alcoholics recovering substantially (Reed, Grant, & Rourke, 1992). These staff people also know, intuitively and explicitly, that clients will exhibit mild difficulties in absorbing, processing, and using new information and experience, and they can adjust their expectations and inputs appropriately.

The more serious cognitive disorders require careful upfront assessment to determine the best treatment approach. A person with severe cognitive impairment who requires continual and constant supervision makes the issue of dual diagnosis treatment irrelevant. The caretaker (preferably one without a chemical use problem) can ensure abstinence by stopping access. Moderate impairment, where the individual requires some supervision, almost always requires dual diagnosis treatment. Mild to moderate impairment (where judgment remains relatively intact, the capacity for independent living remains, and the performance of self-care activities is adequate, but where there are work and social difficulties) requires evaluation regarding impulse control and ability to learn at reasonable rates and with standard procedures to determine the need for dual diagnosis treatment. Serious learning difficulties and/or poor impulse control suggest the need for specialized treatment.

Other considerations for treatment planning are the history and course of the disorder. Especially for younger persons, recovery from traumatic head injuries can be substantial. Abstinence from alcohol often results in at least the partial return of cognitive abilities. On the other hand, a rapidly progressive dementia such as early-onset Alzheimers makes investment of time, energy, and resources in chemical dependency treatment questionable. A good rule of thumb is to determine the rate of improvement or deterioration over a 6-month period and to expect little additional improvement after 1 year. To repeat, abstinence is essential if any improvement is to occur.

Consequently, we like to inquire about the following to determine the need for specialized dual diagnosis treatment: the exact diagnosis of the cognitive disorder, if known; the ability to provide self-care; the capacity for independent living; impulse control problems such as tantrums and assaultiveness; the ability to take direction; response to new situations and material; the change in mental status over at least 6 months, if applicable; response to previous rehabilitation efforts; the level of functioning prior to the onset of the cognitive disorder; and the availability of supervised living situations. We combine these data to make a determination of a client's treatment needs and potential for successful treatment.

Neuropsychological testing can be of invaluable assistance in assessing the general level of cognitive functioning as well as in pinpointing specific deficits and capabilities. Clients also appreciate an honest, factually based explanation of their difficulties in functioning. We tailor our material to make use of any strengths that the client has in visual–motor or auditory–verbal modalities. Neuropsychological tests might have different interpretations among the dually diagnosed, and a psychologist with appropriate experience will hopefully be available (Carpenter & Hittner, 1997). Personality testing can also pinpoint emotional issues likely to interfere with treatment, such as hopelessness, passivity, or disinhibition. Pilot investigations of cognitive rehabilitation strategies have trained chronic alcohol abusers on various cognitive tests and shown generalization to new tasks, but these remain experimental at this point (Allen, Goldstein, & Seaton, 1997).

We generally recommend the use of medications with cognitive disorders only when it is subject to careful assessment and monitoring. Medication, especially at high levels, can increase confusion and agitation. Antipsychotic medications can be useful with psychotic symptoms or emotional lability, as can antiseizure medication. A seizure disorder requires antiseizure medication. We do try to determine whether the seizures were secondary to alcohol or other sedative withdrawal and not correctly diagnosed at the time. We have also seen a few individuals abuse the seizure medication Phenobarbitol (especially where they have abused alcohol or the benzodiazepines and then experience difficulty obtaining these preferred chemicals). Use of seizure medications with the potential dually diagnosed client requires careful evaluation and monitoring. Antidepressants are also helpful for the major depressions commonly experienced by these clients, but again need careful monitoring by a medical professsional.

We use many of the same general interventions for these clients that we would use for the person suffering from schizophrenia. Prompts and praise from staff are useful, as are the use of cuing devices such as checklists, reminder cards, and daily schedules. Keeping material simple and concrete, repeating material frequently, and applying new material and practicing new behavior on a situation-by-situation basis are also useful. Watch out for the talks-good-but-can't-apply-it syndrome. Some clients with subtle dementias still have intact verbal skills but cannot generalize concepts or have learned to fake normality in superficial interactions. Test them for comprehension and performance by asking them to repeat back summaries of information, to give examples, and so forth. We use audiotapes for those with reading and writing difficulties and movies and role playing for those with auditory–verbal problems. We supplement this treatment with skills training and educational/vocational assistance where needed. We also do grief work around the client's losses and build damaged egos by identifying strengths and providing opportunities for success.

Substance Disorder Counseling

Abstinence is the only goal for the person with a cognitive disorder. A brain especially vulnerable to the toxic effects of chemicals and compromised in its abilities does not need more of the same.

Stepwork needs to be concrete and simple. We use flash cards and simple one-line questions and answers with this group. Generally the stepwork we use with the schizophrenic individual is most useful with this group (see Appendix 1). These clients can participate fully in Alcoholics Anonymous meetings. They may need a support person to accompany them to meetings and assure that they arrive in the right location. The support person can also help prevent rambling and incoherent comments during the meeting. Nonverbal as well as verbal cuing on the part of the counselor can condition the client to develop good group behavior. Some clients with dementia may never completely get to the highest philosophical level of development in the program, but even the simple behavioral prescriptions of AA such as "put a plug in the jug" and the all-purpose prescription of "go to a meeting" provide reinforcement of the message to do something other than drink. Other strategies to ease entry into 12-step fellowships with these clients include going first to speaker meetings, allowing clients to refrain from speaking, and introducing clients to AA slogans and language prior to meetings (Kramer & Hoisington, 1992). Attendance at AA can also provide a social support system of persons often sympathetic to and used to interacting with those with various forms of alcohol-induced dementia.

Corrigan, Lamb-Hart, and Rust (1995) describe a model program for persons with dementia and a substance abuse disorder with encouraging outcome data. Key aspects of the program included active case management and a team approach; comprehensive assessment, including neuropsychological assessment; pretreatment education groups to enhance motivation for sobriety and an ongoing alcohol and drug group; a special 12-step meeting specifically designed for their clients; and vocational counseling.

Relapse Prevention

Relapse issues with this group of clients are similar to those encountered in working with schizophrenics. Demoralization and the loss of structured roles increase the allure of chemicals and the time available for substance use and thus need to be addressed.

Prognosis for this group depends on the particular disorder and its severity. We have had some successes where we have carefully tailored our approach to the specific individual and provided intensive structured aftercare arrangements. It is above all important to remember not to fall into the trap of whether or not these clients are truly alcoholic. *Any* use of alcohol or drugs in this population will only add to deterioration of what functional thinking they possess. Therefore, the counselor should view any use as problematic, and a dual diagnosis approach, with abstinence as the goal, is the treatment of choice.

CHAPTER 7

The Affective and Anxiety Disorders

Suicide would be a step up from how I feel; it would
require a plan!
      —Bob E., a member of a 12-step program

Dual recovery for clients with one of the affective disorders (bipolar disorder and major depression) or the anxiety disorders is the focus of this
chapter. We have included a discussion of attention deficit disorder
under that of bipolar disorder for reasons discussed below. This chapter
follows the same format as the preceding one. All diagnostic criteria and
most of the information on prognosis are again from DSM-IV except
where there are separate citations (see American Psychiatric Association,
1994). We have also included examples of treatment plans and, in Appendix 1, examples of special stepwork for each set of diagnoses.

CLIENTS WITH BIPOLAR DISORDER
Diagnostic Features

Bipolar disorder is the more recent term for manic depression. The cardinal feature of a bipolar disorder is a distinct period of extreme swings
of mood and behavior ranging from manic euphoria and hyperactivity
to depressed sadness and immobility. Some clients have only manic episodes, but most will have a history of both kinds of swings or will go on
to have both. In addition, some clients will appear for treatment only
during depressed episodes because they enjoy the highs too much or
because the highs are only mild (hypomania) and do not lead to major
difficulties. DSM-IV (American Psychiatric Association, 1994) outlines
several criteria for a manic episode as well as several subtypes of bipolar
disorder. The first criterion for bipolar disorder is a distinct period of
abnormal and persistently elevated, expansive, or irritable mood lasting
at least 1 week. The person must also exhibit three or more of the fol-

lowing symptoms: (1) inflated self-esteem; (2) decreased need for sleep; (3) greater talkativeness than usual or pressure to keep talking; (4) flight of ideas or racing thoughts; (5) distractibility; (6) increase in goal-directed activity or psychomotor agitation; and (7) excessive involvement in pleasurable activities that potentially have negative consequences such as buying sprees or promiscuity.

Bipolar I type refers to classic manic–depressive illness. Bipolar II type involves a history of one or more episodes of major depression accompanied by at least one hypomanic episode. Hypomania is defined by the symptoms of an elevated mood for at least 4 days and three of the symptoms listed above for mania. We are always careful to assess for hypomania in clients with a history of recurrent major depressions in order to rule out bipolar disorder, type II. Bipolar I disorder tends to be a recurrent illness, and, while the majority of individuals return to normal functioning between episodes, 20–30% tend to show residual symptoms. A small percentage of individuals with bipolar disorder, particularly women, qualify for the specifier of rapid cycling bipolar disorder, when four or more episodes of mood disturbance occur in the preceding 12 months. People with bipolar disease can become psychotic and be misdiagnosed as suffering from schizophrenia. In our experience adolescents who are acting out can also be undiagnosed bipolars. The energy by which some antisocial adolescents propel themselves into trouble often turns out to be a manic episode that is treatable with medication. Table 4 references key symptoms and problems for the manic phase. (See Table 5 in the section on major depresssion for symptoms and problems for the depressed phase.

Key Treatment Issues

People suffering from bipolar disease present three key treatment issues. First is medication compliance. Bipolar disorder is a disorder of brain chemistry and the drugs Neurontin (gabapentin), Depakote (divalproex), Tegretol (carbamazepine), or Eskalith (lithium carbonate) control the symptoms in at least 40–60% of the cases (Thase & Kupfer, 1996). Sometimes medical professionals supplement these medications with an antipsychotic during the acute phase or employ an antidepressant or a combination of antimanic agents. However, many bipolar clients like the highs (while they dread the lows) and often stop taking their medications. Another refrain we have heard is that they had been taking their medications, that they were doing just fine, and then decided that they did not need them! Finally, people on most of these medications require routine blood tests to ascertain blood levels and to monitor for toxic side effects. This is annoying and can be a constant reminder of their "ab-

TABLE 4. Mania

Feeling	Thinking	Behavior	Interpersonal relations and role functioning
Euphoric, up, high	Grandiose, unrealistically optimistic	Hyperactive	Conflict with family, authority, anyone saying no
Often irritable, angry, especially when blocked		Decreased sleep	
	Racing thoughts	Flamboyant, loud, outrageous manner	Decreased functioning during acute episodes
	Distractible	Many projects, reckless activity	
	Confused in severe cases		Often good functioning between episodes
	Poor problem solving		
	Greater impairment of visual–motor modalities		

normality." Side effects can also be troubling and a reason for discontinuing medication. Unfortunately, discontinuing preventative medication may result in future medication-resistant episodes (Post, 1990).

Periods of stress can trigger further manic–depressive episodes, even when the client is taking medication. Consequently, the third issue is the need for a balanced lifestyle, with a reasonable mixture of work, play, love, and proper attention to nutrition and exercise. Also helpful is client use of stress management and time management skills. The counselor can make these a focus of treatment once the client is stable. Research studies have indicated value in follow-up supportive psychotherapy for major depression (Thase & Kupfer, 1996). There is no research to support—but also no reason not to believe—that this is also helpful for those with bipolar disorder.

Individuals with bipolar disease are at increased risk to abuse, or become dependent on, chemicals. The ECA Study found a lifetime prevalence rate of 60.7% and a risk ratio of 11 times greater than the average person (Regier et al., 1990). The National Comorbidity Survey found the lifetime prevalence rate for mania among men with alcohol abuse to be 0.3% and for women, 3.8%; among men who are alcohol dependent it was 6.2%, versus 6.8% among women (Kessler et al., 1997). Another careful study found evidence for elevated risk of independent bipolar disorder (as well as panic and social phobias) among a large sample of alcoholics seeking treatment (Schuckit, Tipp, & Bucholz, 1997). Mania, like chemical dependency, is a good example of out-of-control behavior, and the two together are an explosive combination. The fact that these individuals accelerate their chemical use during the manic phase has led some to believe that they are engaged in self-medicating (albeit to their detriment) and that therefore controlling the mania will largely eliminate the chemical use problem. The scant research available is mixed on this issue, with some evidence for the independence of each disorder and some indicating that the alcoholism is secondary to, or a trigger for a latent vulnerability to, bipolar illness (Strakowski, McElroy, Keck, & West, 1996; Winokur et al., 1994). We believe that this is not always the case. We have seen people with bipolar disease who cannot stop abusing alcohol or drugs between episodes and whose failure to maintain abstinence contributes to constant manic relapse. Furthermore, a substance use disorder interferes with recovery from the bipolar disorder and contributes to such complications as increased hospitalizations (Strakowski et al., 1996; Feinman & Dunner, 1996). Dually diagnosed bipolar clients may also abuse other psychotropic medications prescribed for them (Weiss, Greenfield, et al., 1998). Consequently, abstinence is the third key issue, since there is a high risk of developing a substance use disorder with all its complications. Monitoring clients' status on an abstinence contract can help to solve the problem of an independent substance use disorder. Monitoring clients' use of prescribed medication is also important.

General Treatment Strategies and Tactics

Alcoholics and other addicts often have faster than average clearance times for medications and may take higher levels of medication to achieve an effect. Conversely, late-stage alcoholics may have lower clearance rates. Making sure that clients follow up on blood tests is important to make sure that they are not suffering severe medical side effects and that they are taking a therapeutic dose of medication.

Education about their illness and the need for medication is often effective in maintaining compliance, but some clients require case-management-type monitoring to help them stay on medications (Parikh et al., 1997). Educating families about the illness, helping members deal with the family members out-of-control behavior, and referral to a support group are very often necessary and helpful (Parikh et al., 1997). Living with a cyclone is not easy. As with schizophrenics, high levels of expressed emotionality in families is a predictor of relapse for the affective disorders (Butzlaff & Hooley, 1998; Honig, Hofman, Rosendaal, & Dingemanns, 1997). Family members benefit from providers' explaining how their ill relative isn't doing "these things on purpose to torture you" and how, "in fact, it has nothing to do with you, really." Applied medical insight is generally helpful in reducing anger and guilt within the family. Coverage of chemical dependence issues is also important.

When the mania is very acute, hospitalization is necessary to stabilize behavior and ensure initial abstinence. Intensive outpatient treatment can be quite effective in both initiating and maintaining sobriety in cases where the manic episode is not so acute. People with bipolar disease can also be treated successfully in a standard chemical dependency program if they have had at least several months of stability on medication, or where psychiatric consultation is available and counseling staff are well versed in working with this population. If not angry and threatening, persons in a manic state can be fun to work with, but only for short periods. Their enthusiasm, energy, and giddy mood are infectious but ultimately tiring. As a general rule, we avoid any attempt to stop the manic behavior. Instead, we try to redirect the energy into such things as taking notes (often copious) during meetings or encouraging fast pacing up and down the hallway. Sometimes lowering stimulation levels with brief timeouts in their room or making sure there is no loud music is useful. We limit the client to 5 minutes of air time in group per comment, permit no more than three air times a group, and require him/her to be seated. We establish hand signals or cue words with the client in order to get him/her to slow down or terminate lengthy or rambling monologues.

While the intense moods and behavior of the person suffering from bipolar disorder grab the most attention, providers should keep in mind that individuals with this disorder can suffer from permanently impaired verbal learning and neurocognitive executive functions such as following a plan and that those persons with both a bipolar disorder and a history of alcohol use are especially impaired (van Gorp, Alshuler, Theberge, Wilkins, & Dixon 1998). The principles used for schizophrenia such as repetition and structure will assist these clients in learning what they need to know and in following plans.

Substance Disorder Counseling

We ask anyone in a manic phase to keep his responses to chemical dependency lectures and stepwork clear, concise, and as reality-based as possible. We respond with gentle but firm limit setting to such things as 50 written pages of run-on sentences, designation of themselves as the Higher Power, and attempts to rewrite the Twelve Steps. As medication levels approach the therapeutic range, these individuals will become more and more workable. The recovery approach can help clients deal not only with their chemical dependency but also their bipolar illness. Both are diseases, both involve issues of out-of-control behavior, and both provide a way of doing grief work and repairing the personal and interpersonal damage associated with these diseases. Examples of stepwork specially intended for the bipolar client can be found in Appendix 1.

We encourage our clients to get involved in AA as well as other 12-step support groups and to get a sponsor. We try to help structure these interactions so that the client learns boundaries and doesn't burn out a well-meaning sponsor with eight phone calls a day or monopolize AA meetings with lengthy rambling speeches on spirituality.

Relapse Prevention

Teaching clients about the early warning signs of relapse and the need to seek increased support and help can forestall relapses (Perry, Tarrier, Moriss, McCarthy, & Limb, 1999; Weiss, Najavits, & Greenfield, 1999). Relapse planning for substance use relapse should especially focus on sensation-seeking and impulsive use. Finding acceptable sources of excitement such as high-activity sports is one way to channel these clients' needs for something to do into more helpful activities than all-weekend parties. "Think-it-through first" drills can short-circuit "do now, think later" lapses in behavior. Checking in with a therapist, case manager, or other trusted party before quitting a job, buying another car, and so forth can help to head off the crises caused by impulsive decisions. Many of these clients are also "addicted" to parties and the social scene. Simply terminating their contact with all others often does not work well. While we would prefer that they socialize at the clean and sober activities offered by AA and other 12-step groups, preparty planning is often necessary with these clients to help them say no to chemicals.

Persons with bipolar disease very often do well, maintaining abstinence and showing few residual deficits from their bipolar disorder.

CLIENTS WITH ATTENTION-DEFICIT/ HYPERACTIVITY DISORDER

We mention attention-deficit/hyperactivity disorder (ADHD) here because its symptoms of inattention and hyperactivity/impulsivity can sometimes resemble mania. To be able to make the diagnosis, some of these symptoms must have been present before the age of 7 years and must be present in two or more settings. Increasing amounts of research continue to support the validity of the ADHD diagnosis, both in children and adults (e.g., Milberger, Biederman, Faraone, Murphy, & Tsuang, 1995). In addition to their school failures, which often result in depression, acting-out behavior, and membership in socially deviant groups, at least half of these children continue to show symptoms of attention deficit disorder and hyperactivity into adulthood (Scubiner et al., 1995). Antisocial and mood and anxiety disorders associated with ADHD increase the risk of substance use disorders, but ADHD also independently increases the risk, with no evidence to support a self-medication hypothesis (Biederman et al., 1995). ADHD is also associated with increased treatment difficulties and worse treatment outcomes among those receiving chemical dependency treatment (e.g., Carroll & Rounsaville, 1993).

The use of stimulant medication such as Ritalin (methylphenidate) or Cylert (pemoline) or Dexedrine (dextroamphetamine) (the generally accepted medical treatments for this disorder) for the dually diagnosed client with ADHD remains controversial. Reports in the literature claim successful use of this medication to control ADHD symptoms in adult clients with a history of chemical abuse and dependency. These reports indicate that there was no relapse or abuse of the prescribed ADHD medicine or of other drugs (Wilens, Biederman, & Spencer, 1996; Scubiner et al., 1995).

In our experience, a careful assessment of the validity of the ADHD diagnosis is certainly warranted. The criterion that the disorder must be evident before the age of 7 is helpful in ruling an ADHD diagnosis in or out, especially for someone who suddenly seems "inattentive" at age 14. We have heard too many stories from our adolescent clients relating how they underwent psychological testing while loaded on cannabis to accept at face value a sudden onset of the disorder at this tender age. In fact, many school districts are now requiring a comprehensive drug/alcohol assessment before completing assessment for ADHD. Memory and concentration difficulties, short-term memory loss, and difficulties in learning new information are common among drug-dependent youth. A urinalysis can be helpful in determining whether part of the problem might be due to chronic pot smoking versus textbook ADHD symptoms. With increased public education and controversy about ADHD we have seen a number of adults who think that they may have ADHD. A careful assessment (including psychological testing) often shows that they are suffering from a major depression, an anxiety disorder, or even postacute withdrawal symptoms.

If the youth or adult is also suffering from the disease of addiction, then the use of stimulants should be avoided. Even professionals strongly in favor of stimulant treatment for ADHD in general rule out the use of stimulants for clients with acute substance abuse problems (Pliszka, Carlson, & Swanson, 1999, p. 101). Even if the individual is taking the medication as prescribed, the biology of the addiction is such that any exposure to a mood-altering chemical can trigger the disease of addiction, causing increased tolerance, personality change, and other symptoms of addiction. The fact that there are effective alternatives further supports a well-founded reluctance to use stimulants. We prefer to use trials of antidepressant medications because they have been shown to be as effective in ameliorating the condition without the potential abuse risk, together with behavioral interventions (Pliszka et al., 1999; Wilens, Biederman, Spencer, & Prince, 1995). Only in very rare and severe cases and after these other interventions have failed do we consider referring for evaluation a prescription for stimulant medication. We supplement this prescription with extensive counseling of clients regarding the risks to their sobriety of using this medication.

Another issue that requires work with adults who are not antisocial is the amelioration of the enormous shame acquired over the years of poor grades, lectures to just try harder, failed jobs, and so forth. The dually disordered person with ADHD also needs to be well informed and educated about not only their disease of addiction but also ADHD. Having a client read any of the many books now available on ADHD is helpful here. Using the stepwork for bipolar disorder will work just fine, substituting ADHD for bipolar disorder.

CLIENTS WITH MAJOR DEPRESSION
Diagnostic Features

The cardinal feature of a major depression is a deeply sad, "down," or irritable mood, accompanied by other symptoms and problems, that lasts at least 2 weeks. DSM-IV indicates that five (or more) additional symptoms are needed to make the diagnosis, including either number 1 or 2 of the following: (1) a depressed or irritable mood most of the day, nearly every day; (2) markedly diminished interest or pleasure; (3) significant weight loss while not dieting or (conversely) significant weight gain; (4) insomnia or hypersomnia; (5) psychomotor agitation or retardation nearly every day; (6) fatigue or loss of energy nearly every day; (7) feelings of worthlessness or excessive or inappropriate guilt; (8) diminished ability to think or concentrate, or indecisiveness; and (9) recurrent thoughts of death, recurrent suicidal ideation without a specific plan, or a suicide attempt or a specific plan for committing suicide. Major depression differs from grief or sadness owing to the death of a loved one unless the symptoms of bereavement are extreme or last more than 2 months. Nor does major depression involve a discrete one-time response to a stressor such as losing a job unless it subsequently satisfies the criteria necessary for making a diagnosis of "clinical" depression. Table 5 outlines typical symptoms and problems associated with major depression.

Dysthymia is a chronic low-grade depression. Diagnostic criteria include a depressed or irritable mood for most of the day, for more days than not, for at least 2 years as well as two (or more) of the following: (1) poor appetite or overeating; (2) insomnia or hypersomnia; (3) low-

TABLE 5. Major Depression

Feeling	Thinking	Behavior	Interpersonal relations and role functioning
"Down," "blue," "sad," "dead" Often irritable	Diminished ability to concentrate, make decisions, solve problems	Apathetic and slowed pace, decreased level of activity	Withdrawn, isolated Decreased functioning and activity
	Helpless/hopeless/ worthless mind-set	May have decreased eating and sleeping, occasionally increased eating and sleeping	
	Guilty feelings		
	Thoughts of death and dying, self-harm		
	May have delusions in severe cases	May be agitated	
	Preoccupation with past	In some adolescents, acting out	
	In some older clients, serious confusion		
	Greater impairment in visual–motor modalities		

energy or fatigued condition; (4) low self-esteem; (5) poor concentration or difficulty making decisions; and (6) feelings of hopelessness. Also, there should not have been any episode of major depression during the 2-year period, a situation that suggests that the symptoms are of a major depression, in partial remission. It is not uncommon for individuals to have both dysthymia and superimposed episodes of major depression.

The ECA Study demonstrated that approximately one-third of those with a lifetime history of major depression also had a lifetime history of a substance use disorder (Regier et al., 1990). The National Comorbidity Survey found that 24.% of men and 48.5% of women who had a lifetime history of alcohol dependence also had a lifetime history of major depression (Kessler et al., 1997). More recent epidemiological research indicated that, among those with a drug use disorder (excluding alcohol) during the preceding year, 18.7% were experiencing a major depression, and among those with a major depression during the preceding year, 8.6% had a drug use disorder (Grant, 1995). Comorbidity rates in treatment centers are even higher. Depending on the study and population, between 5% and 28% of cocaine addicts have been diagnosed with current major depression, and as many as 80% of persons with alcohol problems complain of depressive symptoms (Schuckit, Tipp, Bergman, et al., 1997; Weiss, Mirin, & Griffin, 1992).

Key Treatment Issues

Physiological toxicity and depletion and a life increasingly out of control and littered with losses would tend to make any person depressed. In fact, this "reactive" depression is also often a source of motivation for change and for seeking treatment. Abstinence and a recovery program typically result in alleviation of this kind of depression within 4 weeks (Brown et al., 1995). However, those with substance use disorders are likely to have many of the predisposing factors for developing a major depression. Large-scale prospective research has identified factors likely to be causally linked to the development of major depression. These include: low self-esteem, chronic stress, and severely threatening life events, (with dissatisfaction with family and job being especially stressful); a positive family history of major depression; the perception of having no control in one's life; external attributions for positive and negative events; and sleep abnormalities, as measured on EEGs (Kupfer & Frank, 1997; Rosenbaum, Lewinsohn, & Gotlib, 1996). The research on sleep abnormalities is interesting in that persons with severe abnormalities respond less well to psychotherapy and may warrant a trial of pharmacotherapy (Thase, Simons, & Reynolds, 1996). Some research also suggests that impaired concentration and decision making, especially at work, is an indicator of the need for, and a positive response to, medication (Sotsky et al., 1991). Negative life events not only can trigger a major depression, but a major depression can create negative life events in a vicious cycle (Cui & Vaillant, 1997). Individuals caught in the grip of alcoholism and addiction have stress. Moreover, although research continues and the question still is not completely resolved, alcoholism and major depression may have common genetic/familial linkages (Grant, Hasin, & Dawson, 1996; Lin et al., 1996). Interestingly, rapid eye movement (REM) sleep disturbances at admission and less total sleep time at 2–4 weeks abstinence predicted increased relapse in depressed alcoholics at 3 months more study (Clark et al., 1998).

Some chemically dependent clients, therefore, have a major depression requiring additional attention. Individuals with major depression, for example, who were never alcoholic or no longer alcoholic had twice the rate of recovery from major depression than those who were currently alcoholic over a 10-year period (Mueller et al., 1994). Current major depression appears to be associated with less time to the first relapse and with more relapses (Greenfield et al., 1998). Higher levels of depressive symptoms during treatment are associated with greater urges to use a variety of other substances in high-risk situations (Brown et al., 1998). Depressed alcoholics appear to have a particularly high suicide risk (Cornelius et al., 1995). Current alcohol consumption increases out-patient medical visits but decreases outpatient mental health visits in those with depression and chronic medical illnesses (Jackson, Manning, & Wells, 1995).

General Treatment Strategies and Tactics

There is also good news, at least for those with alcohol dependence and major depression. Studies indicate that, over a 6-month period of time, treatment of the major depression with medication or psychotherapy resulted not only in improvement in the depression but also a lower rate of serious drinking relapses (Greenfield et al., 1998; Cornelius et al., 1997; Brown, Evans, Miller, Burgess, & Mueller, 1997; Mason, Kocsis, Ritvo, & Cutler, 1996; McGrath et al., 1996). An early study showed that antidepressant medication was helpful for those on methadone mainte-nance who also had persisting depression (Woody et al., 1982). In con-trast, one study of depressed cocaine abusers found that both medica-tion for the major depression and relapse prevention for the addiction were helpful but only on the targets of each treatment, with no benefi-cial crossover (Carroll, Nich, & Rounsaville, 1995). In another study, medication had no beneficial impact on any set of symptoms of depressed alcoholic cocaine abusers (Cornelius et al., 1998).

About one-third of persons with an episode of major depression will not fully recover, and those who have two or more episodes are at high risk for having additional episodes. These latter episodes are also less likely to have been preceded by a severe psychosocial stressor. Such data are more and more leading treatment professionals to treat episodes of major depression aggressively and to emphasize maintenance of gains to prevent the development of a recurrent and/or chronic depressive picture caused by recurrent "scarring" that results in permanent depres-sive physiological changes (Kupfer & Frank, 1997). Treatment of major depression is conceptualized now as having acute (6–12 weeks), continu-ation (4–9 months), and maintenance (1 year or more) phases, with the type and timing of interventions matched to these phases (Clarkin, Pilkonis, & Magruder, 1996). Maintenance pharmacotherapy is typically recommended for individuals with a history of three or more depressive episodes, for example (Thase & Kupfer, 1996).

Despite all the studies available, controversy still remains regarding whether medication versus cognitive-behavioral or interpersonal psycho-therapy is the treatment of choice, especially for severely depressed pa-tients, and whether combination treatment is warranted. Our own reading of this literature argues for psychotherapy for mild depressions because it appears to have long-term effects in preventing relapse, combined treatment for moderate to severe depressions, and ongoing maintenance treatment of monthly counseling sessions and medication follow-up as needed (see such sources as DeRubeis, Gelfand, Tang, & Simons, 1999; Thase et al., 1997; Clarkin et al., 1996; and Thase & Kupfer, 1996). We also are quick to make a referral for medication if there is no improvement at all over several weeks when just doing psychotherapy. We also believe that, whether or not treatment for the major depression also influences the outcome for the substance use disorder, alleviation of the current major depression and prevention of any chronicity certainly argues for concomitant treatment of both disorders, with counseling and support groups naturally part of the treatment for the alcoholism/addiction.

When a careful evaluation (including a good history, psychological evaluation, and a 4-week period of abstinence) indicates the presence of symptoms that meet DSM-IV diagnostic criteria for a major depression, the depressed dually diagnosed client should be considered a candidate for antidepressant medication. We always send clients for a medication evaluation who present with serious suicidality or substantial sleep disturbance or significant cognitive difficulties in concentration and memory. The first part of this guideline is mandated by the need to manage the suicide risk. The second and third portions reflect recent research suggesting that these symptoms respond well to pharmacotherapy. Most medical professionals favor the selective serotonin reuptake inhibitors (SSRIs) such as Prozac (fluoxetine) and Zoloft (sertraline) as the first medications to try because they are very safe in overdose, have fewer side effects than other medications, and are easy to use. Newer antidepressants include Effexor (velafaxine) and Serzone (nefazodone). Many SSRI antidepressants cause or contribute to a reduced sex drive, ability to have an orgasm, or to impotence in males. There is also a potential for some weight gain. Monitoring for side effects and assisting clients in working with medical personnel to deal with these issues can help to increase their compliance with the medications regimen.

We are careful to avoid the antidepressants that have sedating qualities or that include antianxiety medication because of the potential for abuse. Psychiatrists familiar with dual diagnosis work have suggested that such antidepressant medications as Adapin, Limbitrol, and Sinequan have some abuse potential, and clinicians report that they have encountered addicts who abuse these types of antidepressant medication. In hundreds of contacts with clients on antidepressant medications, we have personally witnessed only two who appeared to abuse them and then only in a way that suggested psychological dependence. Always consult with a qualified psychiatrist regarding medication issues. Keep in mind that medication can often take several weeks to affect the client's depression, and support through this period is important. Also check to see whether the prescribing medical professional has instructed the client about the hazards of mixing alcohol or other drugs with antidepressants. Clients often report that they have not been informed of these hazards, and not all of them are just seeking excuses for their latest relapse. The savvy counselor, when evaluating for chemical dependency, may also want to ask clients if they have ever reduced or stopped their antidepressant or other prescribed medications before a weekend of drinking to avoid mixing the two.

One way that we determine the interventions needed for the major depression of our clients is to ask them to rate their depression on a scale of 0–10, with 10 the most depressed they ever remember being and 0 hardly depressed at all. We do this not only at the beginning of our work together but also at each meeting. Clients are generally very reliable and valid in making these self-ratings. Scores of 7–10 indicate the need for medication (and safety monitoring, as well). Educating clients about the symptoms of their disease of major depression, permission to be sick, and challenges to shame-based thinking about being weak and so forth are also suitable for this stage. Scores of 4–6 suggest that the behavioral activation strategies of cognitive-behavior therapy and the problem-solving activities directed toward role problems at work and home of interpersonal therapy are appropriate.

Keep in mind that persons with major depression show significant cognitive impairments. This includes slowed thinking, difficulties with problem solving, memory problems, and rapid deterioration in performance in the face of any performance failure (Elliot et al., 1996). Combine this with the cognitive impairments of early addiction recovery, and even highly educated clients are likely to overlook the obvious. Be prepared to engage in some very basic and extensive problem solving with your depressed dually diagnosed clients. Target, in particular, relationship and job issues. Don't accept "tried that already" without careful and detailed questioning of what exactly was said and done with whom. You will often be amazed at what clients haven't tried or have too readily given up on. Write down solutions and tasks and send them along with clients, as well. Contracting for the smallest activity they could possibly do helps to overcome the inertia of depression in this range. We've even had clients call in for 3-minute coaching sessions over the phone to help them move along on a plan of action. Clients self-rating their depression at manageable scores of 3 or lower, in our experience, are ready to examine their depressive thinking patterns more fully. Helping them to distinguish between stress and major depression then becomes a focal point.

The care provider can, for example, gently challenge the reality basis of any remaining cognitive distortions such as "It's all my fault," and "Nothing will ever be better." Helping clients learn how to challenge this thinking also helps prevent depression relapse in the future. We take any increases in the ratings seriously and immediately investigate the trigger and any corresponding relapse into using substances. Readers can easily see that analogous activities addressing the chemical problems are appropriately and easily blended with these interventions.

Symptoms of anxiety very commonly accompany major depression and require attention. Many of the interventions discussed below will be appropriate here. To the extent that major depression represents a multisystem response to stress and involves a set of fears that keeps clients from moving into their future, attention to anxiety is important. In fact, we have often noticed that clients are showing improvement because their depression is decreasing and their anxiety is increasing. If depression says "Why bother?" and if anxiety says "I better stay on top of it all," the anxiety is actually a sign that there is hope building, albeit of a perverse kind. Diminishing the anxiety can accelerate the lifting of the depression.

Building or rebuilding social support systems is a crucial component of treatment for major depressives. Many persons with major depression have family conflicts, and individuals with good support systems seem to weather stress and losses better than those with no one to turn to for material and emotional support. Whether cause or effect or both, an important target for treatment must often be the depressives' impoverished and/or conflicted social support system (Prince & Jacobson, 1995). When marital distress precedes the depression, behavioral marital therapy has been shown to be an effective intervention for the depression (Baucom, Shoham, Mueser, Daiuto, & Stickle, 1998). Other family members will often evidence signs of depression and/or chemical use problems, and dealing with these is necessary. Many depressed people also demonstrate social skill deficits and benefit from such interventions as assertiveness training.

Substance Disorder Counseling

We have found it important not to be too quick to relieve the mild dysphoria of the chemically dependent client that stems from the grief at the losses caused by their use. This mild dysphoria permits a window through denial that momentarily enables the chemically dependent client to see him/herself in a more realistic manner (Wiseman, Souder, & O'Sullivan, 1996). Stepwork and other components of a good recovery program will help to resolve this grief. Needless to say, abstinence is necessary for this to occur. We also monitor for grief that hangs on too long or otherwise deepens into a state that meets the diagnostic criteria for major depression.

A mildly depressed person without the three indicators for medication listed earlier in "General Treatment Strategies and Tactics" who is abusing chemicals may benefit from an exclusively chemical dependency approach. The support network provided by AA, the reframing of the situation provided by the disease concept (sick getting well, not bad getting good), the structured activities of 12-step work, the challenges to "stinkin' thinkin'," the advice to "fake it 'til you make it," and the practice of expressing feelings in a direct, honest manner can all be effective antidotes for moderate depression. Additions would include education about depression and increased attention to faith and hope issues.

Moderate to serious depression requires a dual diagnosis approach. Management of the potential for suicide through contracting for safety, through mobilization of family and friends, or through hospitalization may be required. Medication is necessary. Education about the need for medication and finding AA groups sympathetic to medication usage are both helpful.

We have developed our modified 12-step worksheets for the depressed person (see Appendix 1). In this specialized stepwork we have attempted to assist clients in identifying and overcoming depressed thinking. The hopelessness common to major depression can often lead to a relapse in chemical use. Challenging this thinking and developing a positive attitude of faith and hope are instrumental in building a strong dual recovery program. Faith and hope can be in doubly short supply for these clients. Certainly these clients are often quite skeptical of any improvement, especially when others in treatment get their "pink cloud" (the initial rush of good feeling and optimism that singly diagnosed addicts get early in treatment) while their cloud is still very gray. It is not uncommon to hear very depressed patients even declare that they have been abandoned by their Higher Power, and, if this begins to sound literal, it suggests the possibility of a psychotic depression. Professionals who have not experienced a major depression can often find it difficult to imagine the bedrock-rooted sense of pessimism and inertia that is part of a major depression. *"It's not always denial" is a useful saying to keep in mind when doing dual diagnosis work.* Confrontation or simple bromides and pep talks are not helpful here, either causing clients to think they're really bad or that their counselors are idiots. Communicating an understanding that clients do feel this way is the place to start, as is reframing this as a symptom of the illness of major depression, with known symptoms and treatment, including medication. We explain that clinical depression has many horrible symptoms, including the fact that it takes away a person's sense of hope. This makes sense to depressed clients. Asking clients to allow the treatment plan to unfold and to "fake it 'til you make it" can also be helpful. Predicting that often others will notice some improvement before they feel it inside (a common observation) also helps. Explaining the memory bias of major depression toward the negative can make a review of any positive changes seem less dismissive of their own experience, as recounted to the provider. Frequent reviews of progress are necessary to combat the sense of demoralization. We also put a strong emphasis on strengths and assets and do not allow clients to endlessly castigate themselves over past behaviors but instead refocus them on today, one day at a time and on both their limitations and their strengths. This is especially important when doing Step 4 ("fearless moral inventory") work. Clients in early recovery from addiction often already have very high levels of depression, shame, and maladaptive guilt (Meehan et al., 1996). They often have little or no experience of adaptive guilt that promotes realistic accountability and positive action. In fact, the middle steps (Steps 4–10) are an attempt to train or retrain the recovering alcoholic or addict on "how to do guilt right."

Relapse Prevention

Relapse prevention work should especially focus on hopelessness and fear as triggers. Clients will often fall into a sense of "what's the point" or "don't care" and use again, either because there appears to be no point to sobriety or because they just feel so numb and awful and want some relief. As discussed above, the onset of depression can be in response to ongoing anxiety and fear that seems without end. Helping clients to "let go and let God" and outlining options can circumvent a fear-based relapse. Sleep disturbance and cognitive difficulties are other indicators that can be worked into the relapse prevention plan. Also potent as relapse triggers are relationship difficulties that continue even past early sobriety. We have observed a pattern of low-grade chronic relapses into substance use in persons with residual symptoms of major depression. Typically this is not accompanied by denial about the substance use problem. We do not penalize clients by shaming them or throwing them out of treatment. Nor do we minimize the relapse. Instead we use it as an opportunity to point out one more time that chemical use is not the solution and then work with the client to upgrade or modify his/her program.

The chances of recovery for the clinically depressed dually diagnosed client with appropriate treatment are good. Ironically, the pain of the major depression can actually provide motivation for addressing the substance use and grist for stepwork on unmanageability. The challenge for the treatment provider is determining the appropriate treatment and assuring that the client understands that he/she has *two* diseases: chemical dependency *and* major depression. Abstinence alone will not remove the depression, and psychotherapy and antidepressants alone will not eliminate substance dependence.

CLIENTS WITH ANXIETY DISORDERS
Diagnostic Features

The cardinal features of the anxiety disorders are anxious arousal and avoidance of the anxiety-provoking situation. Table 6 outlines additional features of this set of disorders. Under the rubric of anxiety disorders fall a number of specific conditions. These include: (1) panic disorder with or without agoraphobia (which we will define presently); (2) agoraphobia; (3) social phobia; (4) a specific simple phobia; (5) obsessive–compulsive disorder; (6) posttraumatic stress disorder; (7) acute stress disorder; and (8) generalized anxiety disorder. A useful way of thinking about these disorders is the degree to which there is a specific focus that triggers the anxiety. These triggers can range from specific simple phobias (for example, fear of snakes) through agoraphobia (fear of being in places where escape is difficult or help not available) to recurrent, out-of-the-blue panic attacks up to the anxious-all-the-time feeling of generalized anxiety disorder. The more focused the trigger, the less incapacitating the disorder generally is for the client and the more relevant are specific behavior interventions. The anxiety disorders in general tend to be chronic in half or more of individuals and often have a waxing and waning course. These disorders are associated with abnormal functioning of a number of neural systems, very often of a chronic nature (Johnson & Lydiard, 1995).

The diagnostic criteria for a generalized anxiety disorder include (1) excessive anxiety and worry occurring more days than not for at least 6 months about a number of events or activities; (2) difficulty in controlling the worry; and (3) association of the anxiety and worry with three or more of the following symptoms: restlessness or feeling keyed up or on edge; being easily fatigued; difficulty in concentrating or the mind "going blank"; irritability; muscle tension; and sleep disturbance. Posttraumatic stress disorder involves exposure to a traumatic event characterized by intense fear, horror, or helplessness. The person also goes on to experience a number of symptoms for more than 1 month, including symptoms involving reexperiencing the trauma, such as flashbacks, intrusive memories, and distressing dreams; and a general numbing and avoidance of stimuli associated with the trauma, including amnesia, diminished interest and pleasure, and feeling detached from others. And

TABLE 6. Anxiety Disorders

Feeling	Thinking	Behavior	Interpersonal relations and role functioning
Tension, fear, panic, fearfulness, discomfort	Worry Difficulty in concentrating Preoccupation with future or a threat Narrowed problem solving Flashbacks, intrusive thoughts Blocking of thoughts Greater impairment in auditory modalities	Avoidance of feared situations Rituals, compulsions, clinging Frantic activity followed by exhaustion Hypervigilance Bodily symptoms of tension	Withdrawal, isolation Detachment from others or dependence Decreased role functioning

the person may also have sleep disturbance, irritability, difficulty in concentrating, hypervigilance, and an exaggerated startle response. An acute stress disorder is diagnosed if the person exhibits posttraumatic stress disorder (PTSD) symptoms for only the first month. Panic disorder refers to the experience of recurrent, unexpected panic attacks when at least one of the attacks has been followed by 1 month or more of persistent concern about having additional attacks, or worry about the implications of the attacks, or a significant change in behavior related to the attacks. Panic attack refers to a discrete period of intense fear or discomfort in which four or more of the following symptoms develop abruptly and reach a peak within 10 minutes: heart palpitations or pounding heart; sweating; trembling or shaking; sensations of shortness of breath or smothering; feeling of choking; chest pain or discomfort; nausea or abdominal distress; feeling dizzy or faint; feeling as if things are unreal or being detached from oneself; fear of losing control or going crazy; fear of dying; numbness or a tingling sensation; and chills and hot flushes.

As we have seen earlier, anxiety disorders (especially phobias) are common both in the general population and among substance abusers. The ECA Study found that one-fourth of those with a lifetime anxiety disorder also had a lifetime diagnosis of a substance use disorder (Regier et al., 1990). Rates reached a high of one-third in those with panic disorder or obsessive–compulsive disorder. The National Comorbidity Survey found that 35.8% of men and 60.7% of women who had a lifetime diagnosis of alcohol dependence also had a lifetime diagnosis of an anxiety disorder, with the phobias the most prevalent (Kessler et al., 1997). Among a sample of alcoholics, the concurrent prevalence of phobias was 18%, obsessive–compulsive disorder was 5%, and panic disorder was 10% (Hesselbrock et al., 1985). Another early study found that, among those with anxiety disorders, 15% were diagnosed as alcohol-dependent and an additional 10% reported heavy drinking (Woodruff, Guze, & Clayton, 1972). A recent carefully controlled study of those with alcohol dependence in treatment found evidence for higher rates of independent bipolar, panic, and social phobic disorders (Schuckit, Tipp, Bucholz, et al., 1997). Those with a tendency toward both disorders may have special preexisting vulnerabilities. One study of adolescents found that those with a family history of anxiety disorders had unusually strong startle responses and those with a family history of alcoholism had difficulties in suppressing the startle reflex and habituating to the trigger (Grillon, Dierker, & Merikangas, 1997).

Key Treatment Issues

Abstinence will resolve the anxiety of many substance abusers, but a significant minority appear to have coexisting anxiety disorders (Kranzler, 1996). A comprehensive evaluation to determine the existence of a coexisting anxiety disorder is necessary. At the same time, even moderate alcohol and other substance use can exacerbate anxiety symptoms (Castenada et al., 1996). The use of substances may also interfere with extinguishing fear responses and any new information and behavior that was acquired when taking the chemicals will not transfer over to nondrugged states, the latter phenomenon being known as state-dependent learning (Spiegel & Bruce, 1997). Abstinence would appear to be the desirable goal even for those with anxiety disorders who are just "abusing" chemicals. Incidentally, ask about caffeine intake as well. We have had several clients who had a poor response to standard therapy techniques who turned out to be consuming enormous quantities of coffee.

Not surprisingly, alcohol and the other sedative-hypnotics are commonly abused in this population. Individuals with severe anxiety use substances to seek relief, and this can start the abuse cycle. Taking a drink or tranquilizers "just in case" becomes behavior that reinforces avoidance as well. The converse can also happen. For example, individuals with substance use disorders are at increased risk for traumatic experiences and for developing posttraumatic stress disorder in response to a high-stress traumatic event (Meichenbaum, 1994). Medical personnel unfamiliar with dual diagnosis issues and given distorted information by addicted clients often prescribe antianxiety agents for individuals presenting with these disorders. Even in nonaddicted clients the use of benzodiaze-pines, while effective in the short run, is associated with an elevated risk of rebound anxiety effects in the long term when attempting to discontinue the medication (Davidson, 1997; Spiegel & Bruce, 1997). Certainly in addicted clients the use of such medications after detoxification runs the risk of establishing an addiction, provoking relapse, creating an additional addiction, or setting up the conditions for an accidental overdose because of the crossaddictive and synergistic qualities of these sets of chemicals. Abstinent alcoholic men, for example, were found on a variety of physiological and psychological measures to have enhanced sensitivity to, or be at risk for abuse of, the benzodiazepines alprazolam or diazepam (Ciraulo et al., 1997).

In addition, use of chemicals can promote the false and antithera-peutic assumption that the cure to the distress lies outside of the patients themselves. For example, clients treated with a benzodiazepine and behavior therapy for panic disorder and then discontinued from the medication had worse long-term outcomes than those not taking this medication because of their belief that it was the medication alone that contributed to the reduction of the panic attack (Basoglu et al., 1994). Taking a pill to fix things can become an easy way to avoid work necessary to lead to long-term recovery. Instead, the focus generally needs to be on psychotherapeutic strategies.

General Treatment Strategies and Tactics

Generally we like to teach the person with an anxiety disorder anxiety management skills such as relaxation techniques and "mental hygiene" skills such as identifying and challenging catastrophic fear-based thinking. It is important to teach clients that challenging fear-based thinking does not involve suppression but working through the thoughts (Davies & Clark, 1998; Harvey & Bryant, 1998). Standard interventions for relapse prevention focused on the substance use often emphasize teaching clients these skills, and enhancing this component of relapse prevention is often enough for addressing a concomitant mild anxiety disorder. Aerobic exercise often is beneficial, as is appropriate nutrition emphasizing serotonin-enhancing foods. Moderate to severe anxiety makes clear thinking, remembering, and problem solving difficult (Purcell, Maruff, Kyrios, & Pantelis, 1998; Bremner et al., 1995). Letting clients "borrow the counselor's brain" is therefore also helpful in developing a plan to address sources of stress.

After clients have anxiety management skills, we then move into a gradual, graded exposure to the feared situation and prevention of the avoidance response, a key ingredient in the treatment of these disorders.

For posttraumatic stress disorder, having clients learn to set boundaries and to manage feelings first and then having them work through the traumatic memories in a safe, supportive setting are often helpful. Skills training appears to work best early on, but eventual exposure produces better long-term results (Foa, Rothbaum, Riggs, & Murdock, 1991). Clients with a history of childhood abuse and resulting posttraumatic stress disorder require particular care in implementing their treatment. Readers interested in an extended discussion of these issues and a specific formal treatment model should see Evans and Sullivan (1995) and the discussion of borderline personality disorder in Chapter 8. The provider will also need to assess the family and intervene where needed. Unusual rituals or refusing to leave the home strains even the best of families.

We are also impressed by the high rates of codependency in this population and feel strongly that these issues need to be assessed and treated as necessary. Codependents trying to manage the unmanageable, including an addicted or abusive family member, will be anxious. In fact, our experience suggests that some anxiety disorders, especially if vague in presentation, are really severe examples of codependency. Research on attachment theory has indicated that insecure attachments at an early age are often associated with long-term problems with anxiety (Alexander, 1992). Most of our clients give us family histories consistent with insecure attachments. Consequently, we also strive to help clients learn various self-soothing and self-care skills in the context of a therapeutic relationship that is consistent and reasonably responsive to clients' needs.

We use a kind, gentle, but firm approach to nudge clients with an anxiety disorder one step at a time, one day at a time, forward. Directing these clients to focus and repeating material with checks for comprehension help to deal with concentration difficulties. Unless severely ill, most people can best be treated on an outpatient basis.

We will refer a client for an evaluation for nonaddictive medication whenever symptoms of anxiety are moderate to severe, persistent, and/or not responding to treatment. One way we assess this is to try a standard relaxation exercise during the first meeting. If clients show little response to a relaxation induction, medication might be needed. Reports of persistent, sustained anxiety and/or medium to high anxiety scores on psychological testing after detox may also indicate a possible need for medication. Panic disorder often responds well to treatment with the antidepressant imipramine and clomipramine (as do the other anxiety disorders), and the data for the SSRIs appear promising (Jefferson, 1997; Lydiard et al., 1996). Luckily, the antidepressants, especially the nonsedating ones, appear to have little abuse potential. BuSpar (buspirone), an antianxiety agent, appears to have no abuse potential for alcoholics and to be effective in this population for anxiety symptoms (Ciraulo et al., 1997; Kranzler, 1996). The available evidence also shows that combining cognitive behavior therapy with medication appears to be helpful for panic disorder and that using antidepressants or buspirone, while not always helping, doesn't interfere with psychotherapy effects (Barlow & Lehman, 1996). On the other hand, cognitive behavior therapy appears to be slightly more effective for panic disorder than medication, especially in the long run, for most of the anxiety disorders (Barlow & Lehman, 1996; Rosenbaum, Pollack, & Pollack, 1996). The available evidence in a dual population demonstrated that alcoholics who had severe anxiety taking buspirone in combination with relapse prevention psychotherapy improved outcomes on both anxiety and drinking measures (Kranzler, 1996). Recovering addicts and alcoholics may need higher doses of the antidepressants or other medications because of the increased clearance among alcoholics whose livers have geared up to metabolize foreign substances (Kranzler, 1996).

Substance Disorder Counseling

We have found that chemical dependency counseling with this population requires a particularly well-coordinated team approach. Medical/ psychiatric interventions need to emphasize the need for abstinence and the avoidance of addictive medication. Hearing from a recovery-knowledgeable medical professional that just because a benzodiazepine is legal and prescribed doesn't mean it's OK is helpful for breaking through this particular rationalization. We do want to say, however, that sometimes clients are not informed of the addictive nature of these drugs and may not really know the score here.

Chemical dependency counselors need to recognize the special issues associated with agoraphobia and the panic disorders as well as the other anxiety disorders. Urging clients to attend AA meetings should include an understanding by the counselor of the acute fear of large groups of people that such clients can experience. Avoidance of AA meetings is not necessarily a sign of denial. Small, intimate AA meetings are helpful. In fact, ongoing exposure to treatment groups may even assist in decreasing a social phobia (Egelko & Galanter, 1998). A counselor, sponsor, or supportive family member may want to accompany the person to his/her first few meetings. Stepwork needs to emphasize the interactive aspect of substance abuse and anxiety.

We have developed specialized stepwork with depressed as well as anxiety-disordered persons (see Appendix 1). The concept of powerlessness in Step 1 needs to emphasize the paradox of this step. Being powerless is not the same as being helpless—quite the contrary. Giving up on trying to control what cannot be controlled offers a new emotional freedom and lessens constricted controlling behaviors. By accepting that they are not in control of their drug or alcohol abuse and by accepting that their attempts are to control the uncontrollable are useless, these individuals can begin to make progress. The first three steps of Alcoholics Anonymous can assist the client in letting go of strong control issues and in developing a calmer "what will be will be" attitude accompanied by a sense of faith that occurs in Step 2. This faith can help the person suffering from an anxiety disorder to begin to believe that things will eventually go the way they are supposed to and that "all my worrying does is upset me and it doesn't change people, places, or things." Working the Twelve Steps assists in developing personal responsibility for recovery. One way of demonstrating responsibility is for clients to notify their physicians of their addiction and to inform them of their need for total abstinence from mood-altering chemicals.

Many clients suffering from posttraumatic stress disorder benefit from Steps 4 ("fearless moral inventory") and 5 (admitting to someone "the exact nature of our wrongs"), since these steps allow them to relive and then let go. However, the counselor should go slowly with clients with a history of serious trauma, especially if the trauma was incurred at a young age (see borderline personalities in the next chapter). Many of these persons experience strong emotions and need to take the discussion of remediation at a slow pace.

Relapse Prevention

In our experience, persons with anxiety disorders (especially the more serious ones) are at high risk for relapse. One study found that clients with panic disorders were the ones most likely to continue drinking after treatment (Tomasson & Vaglum, 1996). Many experience residual anxiety symptoms and are tempted to seek relief by renewed use of chemicals or the use of other compulsive behaviors such as shopping or overeating. Working an ongoing program is a key to success for these persons. Fear, anger (especially for those with posttraumatic stress disorder), and stress are particularly strong triggers. Alternatives to relapsing and using chemicals should be simple and well rehearsed in order to be accessible to clients shut down by fear.

CHAPTER 8

Antisocial and Borderline Personality Disorders

If I could just remember,
If I could only say,
Then maybe death would
seem farther away.
—ANONYMOUS
BORDERLINE CLIENT

This chapter focuses on dual diagnosis treatment of clients who have substance abuse disorders and also have antisocial or borderline personality disorders. The latter frequently coexist with chemical abuse and dependency and present great challenges to service providers. All diagnostic criteria are from DSM-IV (American Psychiatric Association, 1994).

THE ACTING-OUT PERSONALITY DISORDERS

Personality is defined as enduring patterns of perceiving, relating to, and thinking about oneself and the world that manifest themselves in a wide range of important situations. Almost everyone has probably acted in an antisocial or borderline manner at one time or another. A personality pattern becomes disordered only when the pattern is inflexible and maladaptive, leads to substantial subjective distress or functional impairment, and characterizes the person's long-term functioning in a variety of situations (American Psychiatric Association, 1994).

The term "acting out" refers to behavioral patterns that have an angry, hostile tone, a mind-set that denies, blames, and justifies, and behavior that is impulsive and violates social conventions regarding appropriate ways to relate to others. These behaviors range in severity from subtle insults to tantrums to physical abuse of self or others. The negative consequences of these behaviors include such things as rejection or retaliation by others, legal charges, or the risk of injury to self or others. The stress of these negative consequences, in turn, can increase the risk of further difficulties such as depression (Daley, Hammen, Davila, & Burge, 1998). All these characteristics make individuals who use acting-out defenses difficult to treat.

DSM-IV (American Psychiatric Association, 1994) defines three clusters of personality disorders, labeled A, B, and C. Individuals with Cluster B personality disorders appear dramatic, emotional, and erratic. Antisocial and borderline personality disorders (along with histrionic and narcissistic ones) are in the B cluster. Writers in the object relations tradition often view all these disorders as stemming from an underlying borderline level of personality disorganization (Svrakic & McCallum, 1991).

The antisocial and borderline personality disorders exhibit this overall pattern and share a number of common characteristics. Anger is a key affect for these individuals and tends to characterize many of their important interactions. All these individuals also tend to report chronic feelings of unhappiness and alienation from others as well as conflicts with authority and family discord, both past and present. Most of these individuals have major control issues, being prone to perceive others as trying to control them and being highly invested in controlling others. They also evidence strong patterns of denial. These individuals are also at high risk for developing chemical dependency (e.g., Busto, Romanch, & Sellers, 1996). When you add the denial and control typically associated with chemical dependency to those same characteristics found in the personality disordered client, you have double denial and strong needs for control.

A third feature of the personality-disordered client is an intense preoccupation with self. It is as though they see the world through a telescope that is being viewed backwards, that is, all behaviors around them or in the world are being interpreted by the personality-disordered clients as being *related to them.* Seeing the world through their own damaged ego, they allow narcissistic projections to run rampant. This sense that other people are intentionally "messing with me" is a feature of these antisocial and borderline clients who are so consumed with self that they literally do not have a sense that many things in the world that occur have nothing to do with them. Their primary ego wound becomes the lens through which these persons view everyone and everything around them. Just as the 3-year-old thinks that it rained "just so I can't go to the park!" the borderline or antisocial client shares this "it is all about me" world view. This ego damage is often what makes it the greatest challenge for these individuals to get and stay clean and sober. In Chapter 5 of the AA *Big Book*, titled "How It Works," this statement appears: "There are those unfortunates who can't grasp this simple program. They are not at fault, they seem to have been born that way. They are constitutionally incapable of getting honest with themselves" (Alcoholics Anonymous, 1976, p. 58) These kinds of individuals who also have the disease of addiction end up with a level of self-centeredness that challenges the ability of even the finest clinician to try to address their self-focused world view. This self-centeredness, coupled with a general lack of empathy for how their own behaviors affect those close to them, is like placing a turbo-charged engine at the command of the negative behavioral characteristics of alcoholics/addicts. It is "self will run riot" (another quote from the *Big Book*) at a massive level. This is not to say that these individuals can't ever achieve recovery, for there are many dually diagnosed recovering people out there. What we are saying is that the personal and spiritual awakening that occurs as a result of diligently working the steps is far less likely to occur in individuals who are unable or unwilling to do the thorough psychological housecleaning that working the 12 steps would imply.

We have, however, worked with many borderline clients who do get and stay sober. Their motivation is not self-actualization so much as it is a primary need to get and stay *safe*. Also persons with antisocial personality disorder are not going to have an easy road to humility or easily follow the advice of their sponsor or other authority figures. They may find that they win at poker when sober, owe less money, and meet lots of members of the opposite sex at meetings if they stay clean and sober in their own recovery program. The motivation for recovery for many to these antisocial clients may not be based on wanting to help mankind or any other motivation we might judge admirable. However, if their behavior has changed, then treatment is successful.

Chemically abusing or dependent individuals also develop acting-out behavior patterns as their disease progresses, and this appears to be especially true for drug abusers as compared to alcoholics (e.g., Schuckit, 1985). For example, the thinking errors discussed in Chapter 4 are characteristic of both chemically dependent individuals and individuals with one of the acting-out personality disorders. Consequently, establishing the diagnosis of a personality disorder in a chemically dependent client must take into account the issues discussed in Chapter 5. For example, individuals with only a chemical use or dependency disorder show improvement with abstinence, while the client with an acting-out personality disorder shows difficulties prior to substance abuse and shows a substantial intensification of all acting-out behaviors and defenses when using (Hesselbrock et al., 1985). Among substance users, early onset of antisocial behavior in one study was especially associated with an increased difficulty in controlling violent behavior and commission of criminal acts (Cacciola, Rutherford, Alterman, & Snider, 1994).

Dysfunctional behavior caused by a brain disease such as schizophrenia has a certain scientific logic that enables providers to think in kinder terms about these mentally ill clients. Personality disorders often strike providers as being different. Why do these individuals act in maladaptive ways? From an objective point of view these ways of relating seem maladaptive. These clients often tempt the provider to attribute malicious motives to these clients, since such behaviors seem deliberate, willful, and/or controllable. Such attributions can lead providers to blame their clients, become frustrated, and lose their objectivity.

We set great stock in understanding the subjective world view of the personality-disordered client. This approach helps us select treatment interventions and remain objective. We find it useful to employ different kinds of circles to represent the person's sense of self and the world. The solidity and overlap of the circles represent the person's sense of boundaries. The size of the circles captures the person's relative sense of power and control of the self versus the world. For example, we would represent the fearful person suffering from a psychotic disorder such as schizophrenia like this:

Self   World

People with a psychotic disorder literally have difficulty in sorting out self and world. They also experience the world as large and overwhelming. Treatment needs to help these individuals firm up their boundaries, separate self and world, and increase their ability to cope. Medication, reality orientation, structure, and skills building all help to achieve these objectives.

People with a neurotic disorder, on the other hand, know the difference between the world and themselves, what is called "being in touch with reality." But they find the world to be a big, frightening place (as depicted in the figure below). Treatment needs to help these individuals master their feelings of anxiety by increasing their sense of empowerment and efficacy in dealing with the world. Such things as assertiveness training, problem solving, and enhanced support systems are helpful for these individuals.

Self   World

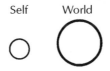

Thus far in our discussion we have emphasized the general similarities of the antisocial and borderline personalities. The remainder of this chapter explores their differences and the differences in dual diagnosis treatment that these disorders require. We make use of circle diagrams to help clarify and explain the written material that we have provided. Table 7 also provides information on the differences between these two disorders and also supplies comparisons with the singly diagnosed alcoholic and the codependent client.

CLIENTS WITH ANTISOCIAL PERSONALITY DISORDER
Diagnostic Features

The essential feature of antisocial personality disorder is a pervasive pattern of disregard for, and violation of, the rights of others—occurring since the age of 15 (American Psychiatric Association, 1994). Three or more of the following are indicators of such a pattern: (1) repeatedly performing acts that are grounds for arrest; (2) lying and conning; (3) impulsivity or failure to plan ahead; (4) irritability and aggressiveness; (5) reckless disregard for the safety of self or others; (6) consistent irresponsibility; and (7) lack of remorse. The diagnosis is more commonly given to males than females. Many juveniles show a progression in their antisocial behavior over time, moving from bullying and annoying others, to physical fighting, to violence such as rape (Loeber & Strouthamer-Loeber, 1998). While the worst aspects of the disorder tend to "burn out" with age, these persons continue to have problems throughout their lives (Paris, 1996).

Key Treatment Issues

The antisocial personality feels little guilt over the trail of wreckage left in his/her wake. Persons with this disorder are exploitative and irresponsible. They lack empathy. Such individuals feel they are never responsible—because it's always someone else's fault or there was a good reason why they did what they did. Maintenance of their inflated sense of self is a prime motivation of the antisocial personality. Looking good, being cool, and being better that anyone else are preoccupations of antisocial personalities. Their image is central to their psychological workings. Having power and control is also a crucial motivator, as is thrill and excitement seeking. Boredom is the enemy of the person with an antisocial personality disorder. Finally, to an antisocial individual, life is a game and the object is to win, preferably in the most exciting, grandiose style possible. Even more importantly, they want others to lose and for the loser to acknowledge this.

TABLE 7. Characteristics of Alcoholics, Codependents, Antisocials, and Borderlines

Affect	World view	Presenting problems	Social functioning	Motivation	Defenses
		Alcoholics			
Guilty/defensive anger	"I've done bad things and I'm upset by that." "I deserve what I get." "Guess I might have to change."	Anxious depression, classic chemical dependency, marital problems	History of adequate achievement, current problems	Self-actualization	Obsessive–compulsive
		Codependents			
Overcontrolled anger	"Look at all I've done to help, and no one appreciates me." "If people would just do as I say, everything would be all right." "I should just kill myself, but who would do the laundry?"	Depression, somatization, substance abuse, relationship conflicts, eating disorders, anxiety	History of adequate achievement, frequently underachieving, fear of success	Belonging, to be loved	Repression
		Antisocials			
Angry intimidation, smooth charm	"If you don't do what I want, you'll be sorry." "I deserve it all." "They're the problem."	Legal difficulties, polysubstance abuse/dependence, parasitic relationships	Episodic achievement	Power, image	Rationalization, projection, ego inflation
		Borderlines			
Angry self-harm, rageful clinging	"I've got to get you before you get me." "I don't deserve to exist." "Help me, help me— but you can't."	Self-harm, weird/regressed thinking and behavior, episodic poly-substance abuse, hot-cold relationships	Episodic achievement	Safety	Clinging, splitting

Antisocial clients sometimes get depressed, even to the point of being suicidal, and may have a history of suicide attempts. This depression is typically in response to getting caught by the police or otherwise suffering the negative consequences of their behavior. This depression is also brief and will pass as the individual with an antisocial personality disorder regroups and redefines the problem as everyone else's. Needless to say, work and legal problems are common, as are marital and family difficulties. Generally it's a significant other who has reason for complaint. Antisocial personalities are just fine with a relationship so long as the other person meets their needs and does not dare presume to want anything in return.

The self–world relationship of the antisocial person looks like this:

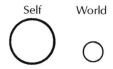

Boundaries are firm—perhaps too firm—and the antisocial is very clear on the difference between self and world. Such individuals believe both that they are more important and powerful than the world and that they intend to stay that way. Empowering the antisocial using methods of therapy traditionally used with neurotics is not appropriate. There is likely to be no change, and in fact you may have simply created someone now better at using the language of therapy to con others.

A combination of biological, psychological, and social factors seems to be involved in the etiology of antisocial personality disorder. For example, individuals with antisocial personality disorder tend to have low levels of brain serotonin (a condition associated with impulsivity) and high levels of brain monoamines (associated with behavioral activation) (Loeber & Stouthamer-Loeber, 1998) Those with this disorder also tend to fail to develop conditioned fear responses (Newman, Kosson, & Patterson, 1992). Early onset of conduct disorder and a diagnosis of ADHD both appear to increase the risk of having adult antisocial personality disorder (American Psychiatric Association, 1994). A history of abuse or neglect and unstable parenting or inconsistent parental discipline due to family alcoholism, loss of a parent, or other reasons is associated with increased risk of developing this disorder (Paris, 1996). While environment is important, a coexisting genetic predisposition is necessary to fully result in antisocial behavior and associated conditions of aggressivity and substance abuse (Cadoret, Yates, Troughton, Woodworth & Stewart, 1995). Genetic influences are more important for adults than for juveniles exhibiting antisocial behavior suggesting more hope for intervening with youth (Lyons et al., 1995). Neuropsychological tests show that those with a personal history of antisocial personality disorder have a deficiency in higher-level verbal skills that may impair their ability to regulate their own behavior through verbal mediation (Gillen & Hesselbrock, 1992). However, by the time they hit the provider's office, etiology is of little concern. Moreover, discussion of the "why" can serve to provide the antisocial personality with excuses for his/her behavior and takes the focus off the *individual's* need to be responsible no matter what the "why."

Antisocial personalities (ASPs) are at extremely high risk for chemical dependency, either because of a common or an interacting risk factor (Slutske et al., 1998; Sher & Trull, 1994; Grove et al., 1990; Smith & Newman, 1990). Those with antisocial personality disorder may have higher rates of substance use disorders partly because these individuals are attempting to increase their overall arousal and excitement level (Epstein, Ginsburg, Hesselbrock, & Schwarz, 1994). Apart from the stimulation provided by the chemicals themselves, a lifestyle with the ups and downs of heavy chemical involvement and the money, violence, and criminal status of illegal drug trafficking can be very attractive to the excitement-driven antisocial. Many young antisocials, suspended from school, in conflict with the family, and bored by the thought of working at a fast-food restaurant, associate with marginal groups where drug use and criminal activity are the norm. In turn, chemical use adds gasoline to the fire, reinforcing their distorted, self-centered world view. Furthermore, antisocial substance abusers are likely to show particularly high rates of cognitive impairment as compared to control groups of non-ASP substance users, partially because of a history of greater substance intake and more head injuries (Waldstein, Malloy, Stout, & Longabaugh, 1996). This is likely to further complicate rehabilitation efforts. Antisocial personality disorder also predicts a poor outcome in chemical dependency treatment (Leal, Ziedonis, & Kosten, 1994; Rounsaville, Dolinsky, Babor, & Meyer, 1987).

General Treatment Strategies and Tactics

The standard consensus is that there is no effective treatment for antisocial personality disorder (e.g., Paris, 1996). We think this is too pessimistic an assessment for several reasons. First, we believe that antisocial behavior lies along a continuum and is not a single, discrete entity (e.g., Alterman et al., 1998):

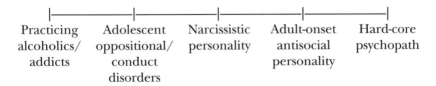

| Practicing alcoholics/ addicts | Adolescent oppositional/ conduct disorders | Narcissistic personality | Adult-onset antisocial personality | Hard-core psychopath |

From least intense to most, we would outline a continuum that starts with *practicing* alcoholics/addicts, then go to adolescent onset oppositional/ conduct-disordered persons, next to narcissistic personality disorder, on to adult-onset antisocial personality disorder and finally to hard-core psychopaths. We do agree that these latter so-called core antisocials are impossible to treat with current approaches. We believe that the others are more treatable. For example, narcissists (whom we sometimes call in jest "sensitive sociopaths") have more capacity for anxiety, attachment, impulse control, and idealization than antisocial personalities, and antisocials low on psychopathy scores seem to be more responsive to fear conditioning (Gacono, Meloy, & Berg, 1992).

Age is also an important determinant of possible success. Intervention in childhood and early adolescence is often effective because the lifestyle is less entrenched and authority figures retain more control (Holland, Moretti, Verlan & Peterson, 1993; Patterson, Reid, & Dishion, 1992). Other antisocials experience a prolonged depressive crisis in their late thirties or their early forties as they burn out and their long-term failure to maintain themselves as king of the mountain sinks in. This provides some motivation for change, although even then *someone else* is usually insisting that the person seek treatment. According to one study, hospitalized ASP alcoholics who also had a mood or anxiety disorder did benefit from antidepressant medication, suggesting that antisocial personality disorder is not necessarily a block to the treatment of coexisting conditions (Penick et al., 1996).

The goal of therapy with the antisocial personality is not to create an empathetic, self-sacrificing individual with guilt. You are unlikely achieve this, at least not early in treatment and not with those further along the continuum. The goal is to adapt the sociopathy so that anti-social clients come to believe that playing by the rules of society can actually make them look better in the long run, giving them greater success and helping them stay out of trouble. The challenge for the provider is to convince antisocial that it is in their best interest to change, as they are making too many mistakes and not operating in their own self-interest. The counselor, then, must chip away at the antisocial's overly inflated sense of self and make the world seem bigger and more important.

The Three C's

The three *C*'s summarize our treatment strategies to use for working with the antisocial personality. You must first *corral* them. Without the walls provided by locked doors and/or legal mandates, most antisocials will generally not stick around for treatment. Don't get fooled by the I-got-caught moment of seeming remorse. This seldom lasts but can be helpful to provide a moment of truth. Even in these cases, someone else with something the antisocial personality wants is most often forcing treatment.

Confront the antisocial personality. Providers need to chip away at their defenses, helping them face how they think about the world and how this really has not gotten them what they want. Remember, antisocial individuals want tangible rewards, not world peace. The thinking errors presented in Chapter 3 provide a useful framework for confronting the process of their thinking and for avoiding power struggles around content. Don't argue the number of legal convictions. Instead, point out the lying by commission, omission, or assent. Do this repeatedly but with a gentle supportive tone. Position yourself in relation to your client as helpful and not as a critical authority figure. We have found it most helpful to begin the session by developing a positive rapport. Discuss with the client what *his/her* goals of counseling are. These might include staying out of jail, getting the spouse off my case, and so forth. Framing goals and suggestions in terms of the client's image is also helpful. For example, you might point out that a smart, cool guy/gal like your client probably doesn't want to end up one of those pot-smoking losers who lie around all the time in shabby little apartments. Instead, you are convinced that a winner like your client would appreciate the importance of being able to give a straight story to a probation officer.

Once you have found a mutual goal, discuss how you might be helpful in assisting him/her in reaching this goal. Establish that the two of you will be working together to achieve the goal by examining thinking patterns of the client that are at the core of the problem. Obtain agreement from the client that he/she wants you to point out mistakes in thinking, or thinking errors that get in the way of achieving his/her goal. Then, when the client is displaying a thinking error such as blaming, minimizing, rationalizing, or lying, point it out without engaging in a power struggle. If the person resists, restate the goals of the treatment contract. If working in a group with these clients, establish the group norm of pointing out each other's thinking errors as helpful peer confrontation. This can be extremely powerful.

The "King Baby" syndrome discussed in AA refers to the self-centeredness due to ego damage of the singly diagnosed alcoholic. This syndrome refers to the puffed-up ego with no true underlying self-esteem. The "I am unique and the center of the universe" perspective is a thinking error that has led many an addict or alcoholic back into their addiction. The King Baby notion is doubly true for antisocial clients and is associated with an "I am everything or I am nothing" world view and needs attention in treatment.

Finally, provide *consequences* for behavior. These consequences need to be immediate, concrete, and to make use of the antisocial's need to look good and feel excited. These individuals do not easily tolerate a delay of gratification. They do not care about what you think unless you can back this up with something real. They are also slow learners who require repeated negative consequences to convince them that it is their behavior that is causing the problem. Use access to activities, visiting privileges, jobs, and other immediate tangible awards. Group contingencies (e.g., all lose privileges if a member fails to exhibit certain behavior) are useful in enlisting other antisocial clients to apply strong peer pressure for prosocial behavior.

Working with parents or spouses about the need to stop enabling and "get out of the way of the crisis" is an important part of allowing these clients to experience feedback from the world that will hopefully enable them to see the world as at least as "big" as they are. Remember that you are likely to find antisocial features and substance use disorders among various family members of these individuals, and proceed accordingly (see Chapter 9 for more on this topic). The codependents want to know "why." We assure them there are many whys but that the real issue is what is to be done today and tomorrow. This helps to get other family members to begin to take more effective action. Educating family members so that they have an intellectual framework for understanding that the identified client thinks, feels, and reacts *differently* than they do is helpful. In many cases, the family members are the real clients because they are the ones invested in getting some help. Furthermore, because of the self-centered and demanding characteristics of these sorts of clients, family members often suffer from high levels of anxiety and depression. The broken promises, lies, and false alibis of active alcoholics, amplified substantially by the characteristics of the antisocial personality, leave many family members feeling as though their lives and feelings have been put through a paper shredder. Family members often exhaust their emotions, time, and financial resources trying to "fix" the antisocial addict. This attempt to control the uncontrollable leaves most family members burnt out, exhausted, and bitter. The lack of responsibility of the personality-disordered addict in owning their own disease or their own recovery has led to lengthy, almost fatal, versions of the blame game. "If you didn't complain so much, maybe I wouldn't drink" is a typical alcoholic excuse given to the family member. Coupled with multitudinous thinking errors for their personality disorder, the combination can leave even the most patient and caring persons feeling used. These sorts of clients establish relationships that are often parasitic. The addicted antisocial will suck the financial and emotional resources of a person dry and then move on to the next "host." Examining the wreckage left in the wake of an antisocial person may often be a highly diagnostic exercise. How many ex-wives have had their cars borrowed and wrecked? How many family members have loaned money that they will never see again? How many loving mothers have had credit cards over-spent? Yet, the significant other invariably ends up pleading, "I am his mother; what should I do—let him die in the street?" In response to this desperate question we follow the motto "to thine own self be true"—inscribed on the sobriety coin (given at AA at 30 days of sobriety and then annually to mark sobriety anniversaries). We give the family member air time in family therapy with the client present so that these issues can be dealt with directly and safely in a therapeutic setting.

Substance Disorder Counseling

During the assessment process assume that very little of the data being provided by the antisocial client is accurate. Let us just say that antisocials are "honesty-challenged"! They have reorganized the external world to fit their own world view. Thus, even though they may think that they are telling you the truth, their lack of insight coupled with massive thinking errors makes their version of the truth a few feet off the chart. That is why—for this population more than any other—collateral contacts and release of information forms signed by the client are a must if treatment is to have any chance of succeeding. It is in the first two sessions that the therapist needs to outline what releases are required, what collaterals must occur. Antisocial clients might balk, but make it clear that you share the same goal, namely, for them to stay clean and not go to jail and so forth. Make it clear to them that that is what must happen if you are to do your job. Do not be concerned whether or not antisocial persons like you. In fact, we often worry if the antisocial person likes us too much! On the other hand, you must have their respect if any therapeutic alliance is to occur, and respect will be won only if you stick to your program. Once you have obtained the agreement to make collateral contacts, be sure that you do so. And do so throughout treatment in order to stay informed and keep the client corraled. Check out everything with collateral contacts, and use urine drug screens and other objective tools. Remember, the telephone can be your valued assistant with these clients. Continued vigilance of this sort must be maintained throughout the treatment period.

Keep in mind the guideline that the issue is not how much of a substance or how often it is used that determines a substance use disorder but rather what happens when the person does use. There is some evidence, for example, that antisocials don't drink as often as other groups of clients but that they do more harm when intoxicated (Longabaugh et al., 1993). Rapid acceleration of antisocial activities when using is a sign to assess for antisocial features.

Even more than with the singly diagnosed addict or alcoholic, the keys to recovery for the antisocial client need to be reiterated over and over. Their defense system and their lower verbal skills makes them "learning disabled," the first because of the deflection of responsibility, the second for obvious reasons. These five keys are (1) don't take the first drink; (2) don't drink between meetings; (3) go to meetings; (4) get a sponsor; and (5) work the steps.

Remind the antisocial client that it is "the first drink that gets you drunk." The saying in the fellowship of AA is "One drink is too many and a thousand is never enough!"

The Twelve Step recovery model can be very effective with these individuals when combined with the strategies outlined above. Step 1 is crucial and gets at a core treatment issue. We insist on surrender by the client. Clients need to understand that they are not in control of either their chemical use or the consequences of use. It is important that antisocial clients learn to identify exactly how their drinking/using behavior is out of control, how they had lost control over their behavior when drinking and using, and how they are powerless. Requiring explicit examples is helpful. We also require clients to identify the thinking errors they use to justify their chemical use and other antisocial behavior. How do you blame, manipulate, lie, and so forth, to justify your use and to control others, and what are the negative consequences for you of that behavior? That is the key treatment focus. We proceed with further stepwork, in a homework assignment and discussion in sessions, always with an eye toward the manifestation of thinking errors. Examples of specialized stepwork for Steps 1–4 are provided in Appendix 1.

Outpatient work with the antisocial personality can be difficult. Outpatient providers by themselves seldom have the external controls needed to enforce compliance. Standard chemical dependency programs usually manage the thinking errors of the chemically dependent individual well, but in our experience the genuine antisocial personality is too disruptive for most chemical dependency programs to treat successfully. Programs with expertise in dealing with antisocials (and the ability to restrain acting out) and with the backup provided by parental consent or court mandates are generally required for success in the early stages of treatment and until acute denial issues have been worked through. In our treatment team review sessions of these clients, we always start with a review of how "tight" the corral is and take active steps to assure that the client is corralled.

Relapse Prevention

Efforts at relapse prevention must be ongoing and often require an ongoing corral to be effective. We typically ask family members, employers, or judges to keep up the surveillance period for as long a time as possible. Key relapse triggers for antisocials are boredom, the need for excitement, and any challenge to their overly high but unstable self-esteem. Finding new, exciting legal activities and more productive sources of self-esteem are helpful.

Remember, antisocials get clean and sober for their own reasons, not your reasons. Go for prorecovery behavior, and do not worry about motivation. It is highly unlikely that antisocials will develop genuine remorse and altruistic reasons for staying clean and sober. However, they may be interested if it will help them win at poker, make more money, or stay out of jail.

CLIENTS WITH BORDERLINE PERSONALITY DISORDER
Diagnostic Features

Borderline personality disorders are a great challenge for the treatment provider. Individuals with borderline personality disorder are semi-permanently unstable, with wide-ranging and persistent instability of self-image, interpersonal relationships, affects, and marked impulsivity. Indicators of this disorder include five or more of the following: (1) frantic efforts to avoid real or imagined abandonment; (2) a patter of unstable and intense interpersonal relationships alternating between extreme idealization and its opposite, devaluation; (3) identity disturbance; (4) impulsivity (not including the next criterion) (5) recurrent suicidal behavior, gestures, threats, or self-mutilating behavior; (6) marked reactivity of mood; (7) chronic feelings of emptiness; (8) intense inappropriate anger or difficulty in controlling anger; (9) transient stress-related paranoid ideation or severe dissociative symptoms. The two symptom domains of interpersonal and identity stability and of impulsivity and affective instability would appear to be the crucial features of the disorder (Blais, Hilsenroth, & Castlebury, 1997). Females make up the majority of diagnosed cases, with rates of 10% of clients in outpatient settings and 20% of patients in psychiatric hospital settings (American Psychiatric Association, 1994).

Key Treatment Issues

There is currently no evidence of direct genetic transmission of borderline personality disorder, although there may be indirect contributions in terms of such things as a genetically based tendency toward interpersonal sensitivity (Figueroa, Silk, Huth, & Lohr, 1997; Torgersen, 1994). Both theoretical speculations and an increasing amount of research in the past decade indicate that a severely dysfunctional family provokes the borderline condition. Physical and sexual abuse, neglect, hostile conflict, and early parental loss or separation are common in the childhood histories of those with borderline personality disorder (American Psychiatric Association, 1994). Most studies have found that borderline personalities have experienced not only emotional neglect but also intense and repeated abuse, especially childhood sexual abuse, with, for example, abuse, dissociation and self-mutilation being highly correlated (Oldham, Skodol, Gallaher, & Kroll, 1996; Silk, Lee, Hill, & Lohr, 1995; Brodsky, Cloiter, & Dulit, 1995; Shearer, 1994; Weaver & Clum, 1993; Links & van Reekum, 1993).

Attachment theory and research has identified a fearful/disorganized type of attachment associated with such borderline-type characteristics as dissociation, unstable and intense affect, poor impulse control, ambivalent relationships, a very negative world view, disorganization, and undirected fear and distress (Gunderson, 1996; Alexander, 1992). Caretaking that is chaotic and fear-inducing produces this type of insecure attachment. Sexual and physical abuse and kidnapping are the childhood traumas most associated with later difficulties, with such traumas independently contributing to later psychiatric disorders above and beyond any general family pathology or preexisting individual symptoms (Boney-McCoy & Finkelhor, 1996).

Early abuse and neglect have also been associated with impaired neurophysiology in general and a chronic state of hyperarousal and a disequilibrium between approach/excitatory and avoidance/inhibitory mind–body systems in particular that produces strong vulnerability to stress (LeDoux, 1996; Galvin et al., 1991; Wilson, 1989). One study, for example, found that a certain type of chemical challenge in persons with borderline personality disorder produced a spacey/high reaction consistent with an impulsive personality disorder and opposite to the reaction of persons with obsessive–compulsive disorders (Stein et al., 1996). Moreover, substantial numbers of persons diagnosed with borderline personality disorder suffer from developmental or acquired cognitive impairments consistent with difficulty in monitoring, organizing, and regulating behavior (van Reekum et al., 1996; Swirsky-Sacchetti et al., 1993).

One way to conceptualize borderline personalities is to consider them as subject to profound, complicated, and chronic kind of posttraumatic stress disorder. Consistent with this formulation, van der Kolk and his colleagues have proposed a syndrome they term "Disorder of Extreme Stress (DES)" for individuals who have experienced prolonged, repetitive, and severe trauma (van der Kolk et al., 1993, cited in Meichenbaum, 1994). DES symptoms include impairment in the regulation of affective arousal; dissociation and amnesia; alterations in self-perception, especially excessive guilt and shame; alterations in relations with others, including trust difficulties; and alterations in systems of meaning, such as despair and hopelessness. Arntz (1994) articulates the view that severe childhood trauma has left clients diagnosed with borderline personality disorder with entrenched beliefs that others are dangerous and malignant and that clients themselves are powerless, vulnerable, bad, and unacceptable. Evans and Sullivan (1995) identified the FAS triad as characteristic of childhood survivors of trauma, with the F standing for fear, the A for abandonment, and the S for shame.

At the core level the borderline client is a deprived, damaged, frag-ile child who was typically traumatized by a very dysfunctional family situ-ation. Ambivalence is the essence of the borderline person's existence. These people desperately seek the love and nurturing they never received as a child. Yet, while reaching out, they also fear they will be abused and abandoned. Those suffering from a borderline personality disorder or-ganize themselves around safety issues, trying—through various safety operations—to balance getting their needs met against the fear of these significant others. These safety operations very often take the form of antisocial defenses, which attempt to combine entanglement with oth-ers with the safety provided by manipulation and acting out. The coun-selor attempting therapeutic closeness and rapport may experience a very intense negative response by the client. Pulling back, however, elicits another intense response from the borderline individual. The on-again, off-again quality of therapy can be very frustrating to the counselor. "Help me, help me—but you can't" is the common message of the borderline client.

The borderline person is crisis-prone and polysymptomatic. Self-harming behavior, unusual thinking with a psychotic-like flavor, eating disorders, and somatic complaints are some of the more common prob-lems. Also common are involvement in abusive relationships and in re-lationships with a hot–cold quality. Quite often the end of such a rela-tionship triggers the crisis. Actions are often self-defeating. Borderlines are typically heavy users of human services but often with little long-term benefit.

The world view of the borderline client looks like this:

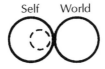

Self   World

The borderline client combines characteristics of the antisocial, neurotic, and psychotic conditions. Antisocial defenses maintain the illusion of firm boundaries and power in the face of an unsafe world. The borderline is quite often angry, manipulative, and self-centered, and exhibits various thinking errors. But underneath this puffed-up veneer is a scared self that feels not only small and powerless but also vulnerable to being overwhelmed by the world. As counselors, we sense the desperate, needy, and terrified element within this person but invariably get enmeshed in his/her defenses.

Just as with the antisocial personality, we also believe that "borderlines" are on a continuum:

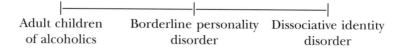

Adult children   Borderline personality   Dissociative identity
of alcoholics   disorder   disorder

Criteria for borderline personality disorder also select patients with high rates of disorders associated with childhood trauma (e.g., Hudziak et al., 1996; Lauer, Black, & Keen, 1993). In our own clinical experience, codependents in a crisis can appear to be borderline but settle down easily and quickly with appropriate support and reassurance. There is no single outcome associated reliably with a history of childhood trauma, and a number of factors appear to modulate the impact of such abuse (Evans & Sullivan, 1995). The continuum starts on the left with patients who grew up in alcoholic or other high-stress families characterized by abandonment and indirect vicarious abuse, and it then proceeds through borderline to dissociative identity disorder, with increasing levels of direct physical and sexual abuse. This progression suggests that all these sorts of clients, and not just clients with borderline personality disorder, would benefit from similar interventions.

General Treatment Strategies and Tactics

Within the framework of borderline personality disorder as a variant of posttraumatic stress disorder, the goal of treatment then becomes to help a victim become a *survivor*. Heavy confrontation of their antisocial defenses and prompting them to recall the trauma in the second session, however, only revictimize these individuals and are not the way to proceed. Over the years we have used the three S's to guide our therapeutic strategies with borderline clients.

The Three S's

We use the three S's of *safety*, *skills*, and *survivor*. The overall goal is to provide *safety* for the person. Lack of safety was the missing experience for this client and is the necessary therapeutic ingredient. A focus on safety addresses the compulsive reenactments (both actual and symbolic) that survivors of trauma exhibit (van der Kolk, 1989). For example, a history of childhood trauma is associated with an increased risk of experiencing additional later traumas, even independent of other risk factors (Boney-McCoy & Finkelhor, 1996; Breslau, Davis, & Andreski, 1995; Dutton, Burghardt, Perrin, Chrestman, & Halle, 1994). Enhancing clients' abilities to be and feel safe in the world is the organizing principle of all our interventions.

In times of crisis, focusing on safety often means *inpatient* treatment as a means of external containment. We have a preference for relatively short stays and specific goals set prior to the admission to avoid regression and further dependence. Kind but firm limits with the explanation of their being necessary for safety are useful for these clients who are out of control and view limit setting as punishment and engulfment. Consistent with other therapists who work with borderline clients, we make extensive use of contracts in general (Allen, 1997). Contracts and other forms of structure that are conducive to consistent, reliable interactions on the part of both the client and the therapist enhance clients' sense of safety and lead to less acting out. These contracts should address such issues as payment arrangements and after-hour and between-session contacts as well as the treatment plan. We use antiharm contracts extensively, sometimes contracting hour by hour in inpatient settings and week by week in outpatient settings.

We help the individual identify and use sources of social support such as a case manager, the crisis line, and groups such as AA. We also help them pinpoint situations or events likely to trigger a self-destructive crisis and plan and practice alternative behaviors. A matter-of-fact message of "we will work together to help you remain safe" is the essence of these interventions. Because borderline persons may have a crisis at any time, we attend to these issues even if the individuals are not currently in a crisis.

The second *S* stands for *skills.* Many persons suffering from a borderline personality disorder never learned basic self-care skills in their family of origin. The lack of good modeling and emotional support as well as the childhood preoccupation with the trauma that they experienced produced a developmental arrest. As we have already noted, these clients are also unusually vulnerable to stresses of all kinds. We like to teach time management skills to assist borderline clients in structuring their days and weeks. Meditation, relaxation, exercise, and other self-soothing skills are important for managing flooding with waves of strong negative emotions when triggered and severe stress responses. We especially like assertiveness training, viewing this as a way to help borderline clients use words and not actions to deal with anger, to learn to say no and to negotiate and protect boundaries (see also Linehan, 1993).

Only when the client has developed ways to maintain safety and has acquired skills do we proceed with *survivor* work. We start at a very intellectual level and avoid expressive, feeling-oriented approaches until much later in treatment. We ask the person to read and attend classes about dysfunctional families and survivor issues. We teach about issues such as secrets and brainwashing and their role in maintaining abuse. Unlike the practice in other groups of classes we give clients permission to control their exposure to these reminders of the trauma by closing the book, leaving class, or switching the topic. As this process continues, we gently and with the explicit consent of the clients question their thinking errors, especially focusing on the role of victim these clients often take. At all times, we take the stance that *safety* is first.

Medication does have an important role to play in the treatment of clients with borderline personality. While no one medication is considered the treatment of choice for this disorder, medications are helpful in addressing such symptoms as impulsivity, severe anxiety, and psychotic thinking (Solof, 1994). One study found that Prozac (fluoxetine) was helpful with anger problems (Salzman et al., 1995). On the other hand, we have noted a paradoxical increase in agitation and anxiety among some of our borderline clients who had started on antidepressants. We use the Minnesota Multiphasic Personality Inventory (MMPI; see Chapter 5) and the scores on various scales to pinpoint pertinent medications for given clients. For example, many of our clients with severe trauma are very energized and impulsive in their anxiety and have high scores on the nine scale of the MMPI and yet are not classically bipolar. Tegretol (carbamazepine) and Depakote (divalproex sodium) have proven useful in helping these clients to tone down affective intensity and behavioral acting out (K. Minkoff, personal communication, 1998). Careful monitoring and avoiding polypharmacy are called for.

Dissociation is an important symptom associated with borderline personality disorder and other trauma-based syndromes (Evans & Sullivan, 1995). When fight-or-flight defenses are not available in a traumatic situation, the "freeze" defense of dissociation comes into play. Dissociation is the splitting off from awareness/control of behavior (B), affect (A), sensation (S), and/or knowledge (K) (BASK; Braun, 1988). The standard PTSD symptoms of numbing/flooding, flashbacks, and amnesia/intrusive memories are signs of dissociation and of the failure of dissociation, coupled with the physiological impact of trauma. Clients' reports of losses of time, of feeling small or young, and of referring to self with different names are signs of possible dissociation. Clinicians might observe in sessions the following signs of dissociation (assuming that the client is not intoxicated or in withdrawal): prolonged break in eye contact, fixed or darting eyes; shallow, rapid, constricted breathing; tight, repetitive, or young-sounding voice; a rigid, guarded, or "fleeing" posture, and spacey, flooding with strong feelings or numbed affect. Treatment professionals need to be prepared to move quickly to contain acute flooding and flashbacks. Simple grounding techniques that reorient clients, such as stating "look at me and breathe," are helpful here. Clients who are dissociated and "checked out" in sessions or classes will not absorb new information or attitudes. Clients may also have a difficult time remembering material outside the treatment setting. Clinicians are well advised to make sure that clients are "present" in sessions and to take special care to make use of written reminders, tapes of sessions, notes, and the like that clients can access outside of sessions.

Managing various kinds of self-harm such as self-mutilation and suicidal thinking and gestures is a particular challenge for those treating borderline clients. Keeping in mind that these clients are survivors and not "bad borderlines" helps to maintain a more therapeutic attitude. Understanding that self-mutilation is an effective means of stopping the pain of a dissociated flashback or of a flood of negative feelings also provides a context for seeing the behavior as functional rather than simply bizarre or manipulative. We treat all statements of potential or actual self-harm as being sincere and serious and deserving of attention. We indicate that these thoughts and behaviors are indications that clients are not feeling safe and that they represent a well-intentioned but not helpful way of coping. We then work with the client to identify and use other ways to achieve the same goal. We try simultaneously to validate clients and to begin work to develop other ways to cope. We work with clients to help them answer the question "What are some other things you could do to be more safe?" As with other types of clients, the best predictor of a risk of a current suicide attempt seems to be the number of past attempts (Solof, Lis, Kelly, Cornelius, & Ulrich, 1994).

We attempt to involve the family in treatment as well. About half the time we discover that the client is married to a personality-disordered individual who also has a substance use disorder, and our attempts to intervene are often not successful. The other half of the time the spouse is a codependent who is overwhelmingly grateful to finally understand what's been going on and to receive support.

Substance Disorder Counseling

As with other clients with exposure to trauma, borderline personality-disordered persons are very prone to substance use disorders (e.g., Stewart, 1996). Often coming from families where members (including the perpetrator) used chemicals extensively, sometimes given chemicals as part of the abuse scenario, and generally seeking relief from their psychic pain, those suffering a borderline personality abuse chemicals. These people often present with episodic but intense use of drugs and alcohol. The progression one sees in the classic alcoholic may be difficult to identify because of this pattern of use. Our experience when doing a substance abuse history of persons with a borderline personality is to find periods of heavy use followed by periods of apparent abstinence when the person engaged in another compulsion centering on food, sex, gambling, or involving membership in a cult or participation in an intense love relationship.

Abstinence must absolutely be the goal for the borderline client, since using chemicals is not safe for that person. Substance use is associated with increased symptoms among borderline clients, including self-harm behavior (Links, Helgrave, Mitton, van Reekum, & Patrick, 1995). Substance use dramatically increases the risk of additional trauma and therefore is a form of reenactment. Prior substance use disorders appear to increase the risk of developing trauma-based syndromes in response to traumatic stress, and abuse of chemicals increases the risk of exposure to accidents and physical and sexual assault (Meichenbaum, 1994). Substance use interferes with learning new skills and working through of the trauma (Evans & Sullivan, 1995). We are talking a horrible combination here when we mix borderline pathology with chemical dependence.

Sobriety *equals* safety. This is the bottom line for dual diagnosis counseling with the borderline client. Drug and alcohol counseling strategies should be paired with circumstances where the survivor was "unsafe" when engaging in drinking and using behaviors. Their disease of addiction leads them to unsafe circumstances. Sobriety can keep the survivor safe.

The 12-step recovery model has much to offer in helping addicted borderline clients. Teaching the disease concept of chemical dependency not only reinforces the need for abstinence but combats these clients' negative self-image. The AA notion of sick getting well—not bad getting good—is helpful in working with the good–bad, black–white thinking style of the borderline client. Using the safety frame also helps to circumvent endless arguments about whether clients are "really" chemically dependent since most can agree that using substances has not been and is not likely to be a safe option for them.

The use of autobiographies or the telling of one's story is one of the recovery tools of the self-help movement. In a 12-step meeting, talking in generalities about "what it was like, what happened, and what it is like now" is all part of being a good 12-step member. Borderline clients require some orientation to solution-oriented ways to do this. Staying in the solution and focusing on positive talk of "what it is like now" is more helpful than dark, lengthy, dramatic tales of "what it was like."

Now, we would not be rigorously honest ourselves if we did not comment on some of the unusual and bizarre circumstances that the borderline survivor can find him/herself in while actively working a recovery program. We have counseled people who have had experiences such as being raped in the parking lot of an AA meeting or found a sponsor who was also borderline where they did their invocation of Steps 4 and 5 in a ritual with robes and blood sharing, an episode that seemed more occult based than recovery oriented. Nonetheless, 12-step recovery in our experience is an effective approach with these clients.

When utilizing the Twelve Steps in our counseling setting, we have found certain modifications helpful. When working on Step 1 we have found it important to focus on the *unmanageability* of the alcohol and drug use. The counselor can assist the client in identifying situations and problems that indicate that his/her chemical use was problematic and out of control. The concept of powerlessness will indeed be a major issue. Many survivors relate powerlessness to helplessness. The savvy counselor knows that in fact nothing could be farther from the truth. Powerlessness is a paradox. By admitting that we cannot control the uncontrollable, we are empowered to live a sober and useful life. "Surrender" (a term often used to describe the purpose of Step 1) terrifies these survivors. They view this in a most concrete way as giving up or being overpowered. Counselors can begin by focusing on powerlessness or loss of control over just drugs and alcohol. Later and with much work clients will be able to apply this concept of powerlessness productively to other areas of their lives.

Modifications of other steps are also useful. Step 2, " Came to believe that a power greater than ourselves could restore us to sanity," is in essence a step of faith. With alcoholic clients we attempt to expand on faith and how things are looking up, now that they are abstinent. For persons suffering from borderline personality disorder, faith and a belief in a Higher Power are extremely difficult to achieve. These persons are living life moment to moment. For them to have faith or hope that things will be any different than now is nearly impossible. What we try to do is to take this step with them in small increments. Ask them to discuss how their drinking or using was insane. Ask them to give three examples of positive things that have happened since not using. Ask them to find even small instances of positive events in their life since abstinence. The concept of a Higher Power is difficult for these people and requires a great deal of individualization. Do they believe in God? Do they believe God let them down? When exploring this subject allow them the freedom to say "I feel unsafe or overwhelmed and want to stop for now." It is imperative that some sort of reasonable faith relationship be developed before the counselor or sponsor can move on to another step. Hope and faith are critical in recovery and happy living. No matter how long it takes to develop this concept, it is time well spent!

Step 3 states that we "made a decision to turn our will and our lives over to the care of God, *as we understood Him.*" We work this step with these clients in the same way that we would any client. We try to assist them in learning to let go of obsessional thinking and to stop trying to overcontrol other people, places, and things. Remember to build alternative skills prior to undertaking Step 3. Once borderline addicts can learn to "Let go and let God," a new, remarkable of peace of mind will follow. We often do very simple rituals such as asking the group or individual client to write down something they are having a hard time letting go of; then we might tie these papers to a helium balloon and let it ascend into the sky. Other ideas are burning the papers or saying goodbye and burying them. Most borderline addicts enjoy the symbolism and the drama of such rituals.

We very much prefer to complete Steps 4 and 5 in a safe setting because of the regressions that can occur. Step 4 is made a searching and fearless moral inventory of ourselves. This can be an extremely volatile step for this type of client. Again, if the client has not got a strong foundation of faith and the ability to work the first three steps, then Step 4 should not be initiated. The Step 4 inventory is meant to be a list of both assets and character defects. It is not meant to be a television miniseries or made-for-TV movie. Referring to pages 64 and 65 of the AA *Big Book* (1976) can highlight the need for solution-oriented thinking. There are some sponsors who hand-out a lengthy autobiographical Step 4 that includes a section focusing on sexual behavior, including during childhood. This particular tool is not very helpful to survivors of trauma. This process can flood these people with unmanageable feelings as they recall their trauma. This is a chance for the survivor to set some boundaries around what is safe to share in Step 4. The fourth step is, in fact, not an autobiography. It is simply a list of strengths and harm done to others or ourselves while in the throes of drinking and using. It can be a true gift for survivors to see that their addict selves are not the honorable selves that they want to be in recovery. Readers will find specialized stepwork for the borderline personality in Appendix 1 under the title of "Modified for the Addicted Survivor."

We encourage AA attendance. Persons with a borderline disorder benefit from the access to support that these meetings provide. We do predict to our clients that they might not like a particular meeting and encourage them to be in control of which meetings they attend. We discourage attendance at ACOA (Adult Children of Alcoholics) meetings until later in their recovery. The emphasis on feeling work and relative lack of structure often found at these meetings, although useful for the

ACOA, is not good for the borderline individual and can lead to relapse into drugs or alcohol as well as self-destructive behavior. We also recommend a same-sex sponsor. Sexual boundaries are an issue for many borderlines, and we have seen some unfortunate relationships develop.

We feel strongly that individuals who are both chemically dependent and experience a borderline personality disorder initially require residential or inpatient treatment with a dual diagnosis approach. Treatment of this population requires high levels of structure and staff, special therapy skills, and provisions for responding rapidly to acting out and self-harm. We also feel strongly that any counselor working with these clients must be clearly in touch with his/her own family of origin issues. As part of their survivor skills, these individuals have become exquisitely sensitive to other people's buttons and will skillfully push them. Counselors who are vulnerable to enabling and rescuing, who insist that clients must get well or be considered bad, or who have weak boundaries themselves and who are easily taken advantage of by clients are asking for trouble when they work with this population. Key notions for managing a counseling relationship with a borderline personality-disordered client include a matter-of-fact, here-and-now attitude. We also hope for the best, expect the worst, and settle for what we can get. Although clients with borderline personality disorder can be difficult and a challenge to work with, many of them will improve with a dual diagnosis approach.

Relapse Prevention

Perceived abandonment, lack of support, and fear, as well as getting into a relationship with someone who undermines clients' recoveries either directly, through chemical use, or indirectly, by minimizing the need for an ongoing dual recovery program are common triggers for relapse. Building sober support, learning self-soothing skills, and prevention planning, however, can all help minimize the frequency and extent of relapse. A key issue here is the counselor's ability to withstand the relapses that almost inevitably occur. Collegial support, self-care, and having policies and procedures about relapse and other safety issues in place will help prevent the counselor from becoming discouraged and from being drawn into the crisis counterproductively. Using the treatment framework in this case as well as keeping in mind that clients in this situation are sick, not bad, will also help.

Readers interested in an extended discussion and a more elaborated model for treating addicted survivors of trauma can read Evans and Sullivan (1995). This book contains an extensive review of pertinent literature on trauma and its interaction with addiction and a five-stage model with detailed strategies for treating these clients.

CHAPTER 9

Working with Adolescents

> Some days I feel lost and alone,
> Other days I feel like a Queen on a throne,
> Most days I feel like my life isn't my own.
> —KATIE EVANS

Treating the dually diagnosed adolescent presents a unique challenge to care providers. This chapter focuses on special issues of philosophy, assessment, and treatment that this population poses for the counselor and case manager, especially when a recovery model approach is used. Working with adolescent women who are trauma survivors will receive special attention.

A SPARSE LITERATURE

Counselors attempting to work with dually diagnosed adolescents continue to have far less literature and research to guide their efforts than those who work with dually diagnosed adults. For example, in 1991 the Center for Substance Abuse Treatment (CSAT) published the technical assistance manual *Approaches in the Treatment of Adolescents with Emotional and Substance Abuse Problems* (Fleisch, 1991). Because there was no research literature at the time, the strategy was to give brief descriptions of existing programs. Almost a decade later, the literature has grown a bit but remains sparse.

Cautious extrapolation of interventions developed for adults to adolescents does appear to be warranted. An earlier review of the effectiveness of adolescent substance abuse treatment found that, while there were no significant differences among treatment approaches and that relapses rates were high, treatment was significantly more efficacious than no treatment (Catalano, Hawkins, Wells, Miller, & Brewer, 1990–1991). Given the similar findings for adults discussed in earlier chapters, this is not surprising, and no recent studies contradict this conclusion. In regard to other disorders, selective serotonin reuptake inhibitors (SSRIs) appear to be effective for adolescent depression (Kutcher, 1997). Therapies, especially cognitive-behavioral therapies, are effective for a variety of mental health problems in adolescents, especially for the particular problems targeted and for female clients (Weisz, Weiss, Han, Granger, & Morton, 1995).

The need for simultaneous treatment of coexisting disorders also appears to be true for adolescents. As with adults, preexisting mood and anxiety disorders, borderline personality, and, most especially, conduct disorders increase the rates of later substance use disorders, and comorbidity rates are high among teenagers (Miller-Johnson, Lochman, Coie, Terry, & Hyman, 1998; Stice, Barrera, & Chassin, 1998; Grilo, Becker, Fehon, Edell, & McGlashan, 1996; Grilo et al., 1995; Burke, Burke, & Rae, 1994). At the same time, while comorbidity is high, there is evidence for independence of the two disorders, with a history of the particular disorder a good and separate predictor for problems in the areas of mood or substance abuse disorders (King et al., 1996; Lewinsohn, Gotlib, & Seeley, 1995). Perhaps as many as half of the adolescents with drug and alcohol problems demonstrate delinquent behaviors merely secondary to the substance use disorder, but another half will go on to demonstrate greater substance use problems and antisocial personality (Brown, Gleghorn, Schuckit, Myers, & Mott, 1996). While earlier psychopathology predicts increased risk for substance use disorders, substance use disorders also dramatically increase psychological symptoms and problems sooner or later in life (Newcomb, Scheier, & Bentler, 1993; Johnson & Kaplan, 1990).

TEENS AND THE DUAL RECOVERY MODEL

Strengths of Using the 12-Step Recovery Model

We continue to find it useful to integrate mental health concepts and 12-step recovery models to implement simultaneous treatment for coexisting disorders to help us treat adolescents with dual diagnoses. While also borrowing from cognitive-behavioral tactics, we prefer 12-step approaches for these adolescents for all the reasons that we use them for adults. As discussed in Chapter 3, this treatment framework includes, among other things, the shame-free disease-process rationale for abstinence and the availability of free 12-step support for long-term relapse prevention. We believe that 12-step approaches have additional advantages when it comes to working with dually diagnosed adolescents. Twelve-step support groups provide a set of peers for adolescents, peers committed to sobriety. Letting go of chemical-using peers and finding new clean ones is a difficult but necessary part of adolescents' getting and staying in recovery, dual or otherwise. Twelve-step groups also specifically model and promote a set of prosocial values that adolescents can incorporate, values that contrast with the typical antisocial values of gang and media-based culture. The democratic horizontal structure of 12-step programs is less likely to trigger rebelliousness in adolescents likely to reflexively oppose anything that smacks of hierarchy and authority.

Some Special Concerns

Whereas in Chapter 3 we discussed our general strategy of blending mental health and 12-step approaches and the associated issues in some detail, working with adolescents with dual diagnoses from within such a framework can raise some special concerns. Rather than seeing an adolescent as exhibiting the signs and symptoms of the disease of chemical dependency, one view is that the chemical use is a part of normal adolescent rebellion, a reflection of the emotional turbulence of this age, and part of the search for an identity. Experimentation with chemicals is seen as part and parcel of growing up and as representing the adolescents' attempt to individuate from the family (e.g., Humes & Humphrey, 1994). Influenced by the symptom-of-something-else model of chemical abuse and dependency, someone with this point of view inevitably poses the question: How do you know these adolescents can never drink successfully or smoke pot in moderation, and what about all the other problems they're manifesting? Another concern involves the practice of encouraging the chemically abusing or dependent adolescent to adopt the label of alcoholic or addict and to "surrender." The fear is that these adolescents, seeking to establish a personal identity as part of this stage of their development, will incorporate a seemingly negative concept into their sense of who they are in the world and not be empowered to live out their lives most productively.

Very few adolescents with substance use disorders volunteer for treatment and are usually pressured into it by parents, schools, or probation officers. Consequently, another objection that we've encountered relates to the issue of adolescent consent for treatment. Adolescents deserve the same rights as adults, and sometimes families and cooperating service systems have unjustly locked up or mandated treatment for adolescents and treated them against their will, according to this stance. Adolescents forced into treatment are victims of scapegoating by the family and are being stripped of their rights without due process. A related argument is that, unless the adolescent accepts the need for treatment, therapy will ultimately fail. Finally, some professionals argue that the family conflict often present among members of the adolescent's family system points to the need for working from within a family therapy framework. Taken as an exclusive approach, the priority must then be on putting the parents back in charge, resolving conflicts, and establishing appropriate interactions among family members. The dually diagnosed adolescent's multiple interacting problems often intensify these debates by seeming to provide evidence for all these concerns.

A third objection that we often hear is that treatment will make things worse. One variant of this concern is that the adolescent will be exposed to other adolescents with even worse attitudes and problems and that treatment would merely constitute a training school for delinquency. Places where deleterious contacts might occur include both the treatment center and the 12-step meetings. Another variant is that medication's efficaciousness for adolescents is as yet unproven, entailing uncertain long-term effects, and therefore should not be utilized.

Certainly some adolescents who abuse chemicals go on to be reasonably well adjusted adults with no evidence of a progressive addiction (Wills, McNamara, Vaccaro, & Hirky, 1996). Families of adolescents abusing and dependent on chemicals do sometimes have a history of family problems such as divorce, incest, and parental substance abuse prior to the onset of significant chemical use by their child (Denton & Kampfe, 1994; Hernandez, 1992). Families and service systems have sometimes made the adolescent a scapegoat and trampled on the adolescent's rights. Young people's 12-step meetings *can* be a great place to score some drugs.

Our Position

There are, however, other aspects to these issues. For most adolescents most of the time, life is without significant crises. Moodiness and occasional high jinks are part of this period in life, but anything beyond this is not typical. Moreover, chemical use by adolescents is problematic. Drinking/using and driving are not a good mix—for inexperienced *or* experienced drivers. Marijuana and "speed" can interfere with hormonal and neurological development. This is a crucial issue for adolescents as they progress through a stage of rapid physical maturation and are vulnerable to chemical disruption of normal maturation processes. Youth who abuse chemicals can also experience interference with their emotional and psychological development and, in the research cited above, are at increased risk for the onset of mental health problems. Significant chemical usage interferes with the development of a positive prosocial identity. The involvement with chemicals can lead to an identity crystallized around being a "stoner" and having antisocial values stressing dishonesty, the rip-off, and immediate gratification. Membership in socially marginal groups, failure in school, and conflict at home do not lay a good foundation for future success.

Exploring intimacy is also not possible when under the influence. The adolescent abusing drugs is not available emotionally and is likely to have problems coping with the complexities of establishing and maintaining close relationships. Similarly, adolescents are exploring and integrating their sexuality. Rape while under the influence or by someone under the influence is all too common an experience for young women that we treat. This is hardly a healthy introduction to the joys of responsible sexuality.

For many persons adolescence is a time of intense self-focus. This preoccupation with self produces a narcissism that, thankfully, does pass with time. However, substance use disorders can feed this narcissism and take it to levels that are very problematic. Especially when parents get overly hooked into these chemically stoked narcissistic behaviors, an unfortunate level of conflict can ensue that ends up being detrimental to a smooth unfolding of adolescents' autonomy. The implications of all this? We restate our guideline that *what causes a problem is a problem.* Adolescence in and of itself does not cause problems. Chemical use often does. We would rather be safe than sorry and encourage adolescents to develop chemical-free lifestyles.

Adolescents have rights, including the right to due process, and the adolescent willing to admit having a drug problem is certainly an easier client, if a rare one. However, our laws recognize that adolescents are not adults, and these laws require parental or guardian consent for major decisions such as getting married, entering the armed services, and signing contracts. Society has also determined that adolescents are not yet capable of making mature decisions when it comes to voting or drinking alcohol. Accidents, murders, and acquired immune deficiency syndrome (AIDS) are also complications of chemical involvement even for adolescents. Gangs are a fact of life for today's teens, and drug use and dealing are a primary focus for these gangs. Fourteen-year-olds are shooting each other. Lifestyles involving promiscuity and intravenous drug use can expose a youth to the AIDS virus.

Trying gently to convince a child whose brain is under the influence and who is in denial that he or she needs treatment for addiction is likely to end in failure. Consider also the plight of the parents trying to deal with their out-of-control youngster. The parents of these adolescents are in a double bind. They are responsible for the actions of their children and for their growth and development; yet, some state laws do not allow parents to access mental health or chemical dependency treatment without the child's consent. We are comfortable treating the unwilling adolescent and, consistent with the research on adults, have generally found their ability to attain sobriety and stability equal to that of their peers who entered treatment willingly.

Accepting the label of alcoholic or addict can empower the adolescent in ways not immediately evident. We feel that the initial acceptance of their addiction is demonstrated in their willingness to identify with the recovering addict/alcoholic rubric. Within the recovery framework, youth can come to believe they are sick getting well, not bad getting better. These adolescents gain new relationships with a prosocial group of peers and older, more mature adults through the fellowship of 12-step groups. Youth accepting the label develop ethical and spiritual values that include honesty, conscious contact with a power greater than themselves, and dedication to helping others as part of their 12-step recovery program. Moreover, many of the adolescents that we treat have coexisting conduct disorders involving dealing drugs, carrying weapons, dropping out of school and physically coercing their parents, and traditional notions of empowerment are the last thing that these teens need!

On rare occasions, either because of the young age of a client or a particularly rough milieu in current groups, we will keep a client out of groups and do most of the work individually while trying to hook him/her up with any support groups at school. Generally, however, we try to assure parents that their teens already know all they need to know about drugs and that they are unlikely to learn anything new from their fellow clients.

We will discuss the role of the family in greater depth in the next chapter. Chemical use does cause family conflict or exacerbate existing difficulties. Whether cause, effect, or both, in our experience abstinence is necessary for successful family work and, analogous to the coexisting models, simultaneous treatment of the child and family difficulties is necessary for successful outcomes. Families torn apart by the devastation of a mentally ill substance-abusing youth need time to heal and the guidance and support of a trained family therapist to help them in their own journey of recovery.

ASSESSMENT WITH TEENS

The Need to Rule Out a Substance Use Disorder

Most of the assessment principles discussed in Chapters 4 and 5 are relevant to adolescent assessments. There are, however, issues especially important to keep in mind when assessing adolescents. Adolescents with substance use disorders are seldom honest about their drug use during assessments. Most adolescents are masters of lying by omission, and this is especially so when they face inquiries about such things as their chemical use. Most adolescents arrive in the office under coercion from some external authority. This makes for a less than open, honest, or willing candidate for an interview. You will generally have to assume that the adolescents that you assess are lying, minimizing, and so forth and proceed accordingly.

Keep in mind the high base rates of use among adolescents and how many of these individuals are *not* brought in for an assessment. Given this, anyone who is sent for an assessment is very likely to have a problem. Occasionally some poor kid gets caught the first time he or she sips some alcohol or smokes pot. More often than not, however, the teenager in front of you *does* have a substance use problem. Your job is to demonstrate why this person should *not* have some sort of intervention or treatment.

Doing the Assessment Interview

We find that a straightforward doing-business style works best. Attempts to use current slang or otherwise be cool just look stupid and phony, and a nondirective approach looks weak and lacks credibility. Most of the youth we encounter are looking for someone who respects them and their beliefs and listens to them without judgment or lecturing. Thus, the therapeutic alliance made during the assessment is critical to gleaning any relevant data at all, let alone beginning the process of building motivation.

We start with a joint meeting with the parent, legal guardian, or other responsible adult, insisting whenever possible that an adult accompany the adolescent to the interview. We elicit all parties' understanding of the purpose of the interview and clarify the understanding as needed. At times the responsible adult has lied about the purpose of the interview, and an explosion takes place. Be prepared to move in to soothe the situation and move forward. We then explain the limits of confidentiality. We tell the adolescent that, while we are not going to tell the responsible adult everything that he or she tells us, we do have to report an overall summary and anything that is a safety or health hazard. We explain that if there is anything that they do not want us to repeat, they need to say so and that we reserve the right of final judgment. We then explain that getting a urinalysis is standard procedure and, if there is a balking or outright refusal to comply, explain that we consider no urinalysis to be a dirty urinalysis. Occasionally the parent will raise civil libertarian issues, and we proceed to work these out with the parent after sending the adolescent out of the room. If the adolescent raises these sorts of issues, we just treat it as a thinking error of a smart person. Finally, we explain that we will meet with the adolescent first and then with the parent to give each an opportunity to ask and answer questions and to clarify concerns. We then proceed to question the adolescent alone in a direct, straightforward style. This combination of clear boundaries, respect, and no nonsense often reduces (but does not eliminate) defensiveness.

Helpful Information

Certain information may be helpful in determining whether a substance use disorder exists, and certain questions seem more likely than not to be answered honestly, slipping thorough defensive walls comparatively easily. Smoking cigarettes, besides being a sign of nicotine dependence, appears to be associated with a high risk for subsequent progression to alcohol and marijuana (Duncan, Duncan, & Hops, 1998). The proportion (percentage) of friends who drink and use is a tipoff to peer group use patterns, a key determinant of chemical use in adolescents (Hoffmann, 1995; Steinberg, Fletcher, & Darling, 1994). Low levels of parental monitoring—due, for example, to a single parent having to work two jobs—is also associated with an increased risk of acting-out behavior (Forehand, Miller, Dutra, & Chance, 1997). A general attitude of antipathy toward home and school responsibilities, coupled with an active social life outside the home inconsistent with depression, is a tipoff to possible problematic substance use. We also are alert to our own sense of wanting to fight with the adolescents because of a hostile, blaming attitude and a stream of thinking errors on their part. This is a tipoff to acting-out defenses and signals either a disorder consistent with the specific defenses and/or addiction.

Looking at systems problems is a key way to assess chemical dependency in adolescents. This includes dually diagnosed adolescents. School is an important system because this is a place where adolescents spend up to 7 hours a day, face worklike demands for performance, and find friends. School is a microcosm of society. Teachers often notice the effects of drugs and alcohol on a child's performance and are often the first adults to notice a problem. School personnel have access to rumors and notice a change in friends. Sometimes former friends of the adolescent tell a school counselor that they are concerned. Memory impairment and reduction in abstract thinking are common in the adolescent substance abusers. As use continues, the youth become apathetic and disinterested in studies. They fail to turn in assignments and are ill prepared for tests and reports. They then begin a pattern of tardiness and then absenteeism. Using substances on a school day or at school is something we always consider to be a serious sign of problems.

Extracurricular activities drop off. An athletic child suddenly decides that track is now boring and that all the participants are either jocks or nerds. Or a young thespian may suddenly state unequivocally that drama club is actually quite stupid, after all. Old friends are gradually replaced by new "cool" friends who also are drinking and drug abusing.

Families are, of course, the home system. The drug- or alcohol-abusing adolescents become increasingly uncomfortable in an environment where adults are trying to set limits on their behavior and where adults expect communication and honesty. Family members will note such problematic behaviors as loss of interest in school activities, isolation in room, and money missing from their wallets in the adolescent abusing drugs, including the dually diagnosed adolescent.

Collateral information, then, is important. School officials often develop checklists for identifying the drug-abusing youth and recommending a formal chemical abuse assessment (see Appendix 2, "A School Behavior Checklist" for an example). Appendix 3, titled "A Checklist for Parents," includes a sample home behavior checklist for parents that pinpoints typical problem behaviors.

Ways to Diagnose Dual Disorders

Finding classic signs of chemical dependency can be difficult with adolescents. Although we have seen 11-year-olds requiring alcohol detoxification, dramatic withdrawal symptoms as well as physical problems are relatively uncommon with adolescents. Standard notions of progression are difficult to use as criteria of chemical dependence, as well.

Adolescents often have episodic, bingelike use patterns instead of gradual increases in use. One useful tip to remember is that a youth who is becoming more and more preoccupied with use, and who is expanding the variety of chemicals used, demonstrates a kind of progression. Remember that adolescents can show another kind of rapid progression involving high levels of chemical intake in one session. Peer-influenced games focused on rapid intake, such as chugging shots and "shooting" beers, contribute to this progression in a number of adolescents. An episode of alcohol intoxication or other, similar drug use episode that results in an emergency room visit is a serious sign of problems, either now or in the future. Progression is also evident in increasing role dysfunction as evidenced by deterioration at home or at school.

Adolescents do evidence loss of control with a violation of their rules for use. Asking the question "Have you ever drunk or used more than planned?" is relevant for both adults and adolescents. Adolescents develop their own rules for drinking and using, such as "I'll never use hard drugs." Breaking these rules shows loss of control. Adolescents will also exhibit denial and thinking errors. Blaming others and minimizing problems are two common thinking errors.

The discussion in Chapter 5 about establishing the psychiatric diagnosis for dually diagnosed clients is pertinent to working with dually diagnosed adolescents. Base-rate issues, the ability of chemical use to mimic psychiatric disorders, and the need for a comprehensive assessment all apply to this younger population.

We have found that troubled adolescents tend to express their difficulties through behavior. Adolescents often are still developing their abilities to reason abstractly and to use words to express and deal with their impulses and conflicts. Adolescents also continue to feel dependent on powerful others for their needs and feel conflict about expressing their needs in direct ways. When in trouble, adolescents are more likely than adults to act rather than think and to rebel rather than negotiate. The majority of dually diagnosed adolescents present with some kind of acting-out behavior, no matter what the coexisting disorder. Many dually diagnosed youth harbor deep anger and resentment toward family members and authority figures. Parents—especially those who had been neglectful or abusive—are objects of intense feeling. For youth who act out, defiance of parents, running away, threatening and assaultive behavior, vandalism, and promiscuity are common. Youth who "act in" rather than act out can become self-destructive and suicidal. Many of these adolescents engage in self-mutilating behavior by cutting themselves with knives and razor blades. Using drugs and alcohol further disrupts effective coping and adds fuel to the fire of family dysfunction. The adolescents then gravitate toward peers like themselves who are learning that chemicals kill the pain. And so the problem escalates.

A common assessment dilemma facing the evaluator is distinguishing normal among adolescent behavior, behavioral difficulties resulting from chemical use alone, and the acting out of the antisocial adolescent who is also chemically dependent. Early substance abuse appears common among individuals with an antisocial personality disorder (Miller-Johnson et al., 1998; Grilo et al., 1995; Grilo et al., 1996). Table 8 outlines differences that we have observed among these three groups.

When reviewing the table, the reader will note that the normative behavior of the typical adolescent is greatly intensified in the description of the drug-abusing adolescent. Drug-abusing adolescents begin to manifest life problems such as school problems, family problems, and some legal problems. The substance-abusing youth also begins to display thinking errors such as rationalizing and blaming. These adolescents use these thinking errors to justify their continued use of drugs in spite of growing evidence that drugs are becoming a problem. They feel guilt and remorse over negative and harmful behavior but use drugs and alcohol to rid themselves of emotions. *Antisocial* adolescents, in contrast, do not demonstrate empathy, passion, or remorse.

TABLE 8. Characteristics of the Normal Adolescent, the Drug-Abusing Adolescent, and the Antisocial Adolescent

Area	Normal adolescent	Drug-abusing adolescent	Antisocial adolescent
Affect	Moodiness	Drastic mood swings, guilty anger	Angry and calm, controlling or smooth and charming
World view	"I should be able to do anything I want to." "I feel like I am not as good at things as I would like to be." "If I steal I might get caught; then people would know I'm a thief."	"I've done some bad things and I feel guilty." "If I don't stay on top of things people will find out I'm bad." "I have to to get money, steal; besides, all my friends do it."	"I'm cool and you don't matter unless you have something I want." "It's not bad unless you get caught." "You're a fool and deserve to be ripped off."
Presenting problem	Moodiness, feeling insecure, unliked	School problems, family conflict, change of friends, drastic mood swings, lying, legal problems such as theft, breaking and entering	Violent behavior, violent crimes, rageful outbursts. Family members and others injured amid wreckage in wake of the antisocial
Social functioning	Adequate achievement, positive peer group, interest, or outside hobby	Current problems, things growing progressively worse	Excellent functioning (e.g., class president, in charge of everything, smooth talker) or poor functioning with numerous law violations and volatile relationships
Motivation	Autonomy, peer identification	To return to previous positive functioning, acceptance of peers	To win, be right; control, seek stimulation/excitement short-term
Defenses	Isolation, minimizing blame	Lying, manipulation, increased use of thinking errors	Conning, pure, and continued resort to thinking errors

Their thinking errors are continuous, and their behavior is blatantly antisocial.

Another assessment dilemma for the evaluator is distinguishing between the true antisocial and the borderline personality-disordered adolescent who appears antisocial. Many adolescents who have experienced serious physical and/or sexual abuse at the hands of adults act out as a way to deal with the pain of these experiences and protect themselves from further harm. A history of such abuse is common among adolescents with substance use disorders (Evans & Sullivan, 1995; Hernandez, 1992; Bayatpour, Wells, & Holford, 1992). Readers will find the material discussed in Chapter 7 regarding the antisocial and borderline personality disorders relevant to the task of assessment. A same-sex counselor for females is a must in these cases, since female adolescents are unlikely to report and process sex abuse issues with a male counselor. The recent rise in guns, gangs, and violence means that many adolescents have experienced traumatic incidents and may evidence signs of posttraumatic stress disorder. Also common among adolescents with a substance abuse disorder is a history of suicidal thinking and attempts, and this is important to assess (Deykin & Buka, 1994). A comprehensive assessment will help to make this determination.

Some adolescents have affective or early-onset schizophrenic disorders. These are often difficult to detect, especially when chemical use is also present, but they need to be considered if there are signs and symptoms justifying this concern. Sometimes a carefully monitored trial of medication is the only way to confirm these possibilities, and treatment professionals should consider this if other behavioral interventions have failed. The evaluator trying to determine whether an adolescent abusing chemicals also has a coexisting psychiatric disorder can attend to the quality of the adolescents' presenting problems and associated signs and symptoms. The dually diagnosed adolescent will show more intense problems, and these problems will have a different flavor than the troubles of the adolescent with only a chemical use problem. The damaged antisocial adolescent, for example, will have a history of cruel and very destructive acts even when not intoxicated. These acts may include setting fires and torturing animals. The early-onset adolescent schizophrenic will be socially isolated and not even have drug-using peers and will also show ongoing bizarre thinking and behavior. The dually diagnosed adolescent with a bipolar disorder will show huge mood swings and may exhibit out-of-control outbursts or promiscuity. Psychological testing done by a psychologist who is familiar with dual diagnosis issues can be very valuable in sorting out diagnostic possibilities. Table 9 lists typical presenting problems, signs, and symptoms that we have observed with dually diagnosed adolescents with certain coexisting disorders.

Evaluators also need to be alert to attention deficit disorder (ADD), with or without hyperactivity, and subtle learning disabilities. Adolescents with such deficits are at high risk for problematic chemical use. Besides their impulsivity, their experience of being different and failing in school leave them vulnerable to the seductive call of socially marginal peer groups and the pleasant effects of chemicals. We have seen several cases where "bad boys" suddenly turned around when on the right medication. When adolescents have any history of inhalant use or any long-term use of other chemicals, evaluation for an organic mental disorder is also indicated. Neurological and neuropsychological evaluation can be helpful here in assessing these organic difficulties.

TREATMENT ISSUES

Stepwork

Addicted youth do not respond like adult alcoholics to discussions regarding health, role performance, family, and death. The statement "You will die if you keep drinking" gets the attention of most adult substance abusers. An adolescent substance abuser may respond, "Everyone dies—plus it could take me 20 to 30 more years of partying before that happens!" Counselors need to focus on current instances of negative consequences and instances of negative outcomes likely in the short run. Today and this week are often appropriate time frames. For the adolescent overwhelmed with the idea of never drinking or using again, focusing on one day at a time—abstaining just for today—is useful. The dually diagnosed youth can often acknowledge how much emotional turmoil he/she is in. This affords the counselor the opportunity to point out that drugs are no longer working and to offer sobriety as an option for pain reduction. Step 1's discussion of powerlessness over chemicals requires a great deal of clinical intervention. The grandiosity of youth leaves a built-in defense of denial. However, all alcoholics are grandiose and suffer with issues of power and control. The addicted teen is just more, much more, of the same!

Step 2 with the adolescent presents some special concerns. "Came to believe a power greater than ourselves could restore us to sanity" requires abstract thinking combined with faith, both of which pose difficulties for the adolescent. We work with youth on helping them identify people and situations that indicate that their life is improving since discontinuing alcohol and drug abuse. There is a famous story told around the table of AA meetings that is known as the Eskimo story. This story highlights Step 2's requirement of faith in a Higher Power. We often tell

TABLE 9. Common Signs, Symptoms, and Problems Observed among Certain Groups of Dually Diagnosed Adolescents

Adolescents with a coexisting conduct disorder

Presenting problems

Stealing
Legal violations
Thrill-seeking element in acting out
Arson
Truancy
Fights at school
Failing grades
Problems with authority
Sexually exploitative relationships/sexual offending
Severe family conflict, physical and verbal fighting

Thinking

Chronic use of thinking errors
Intense denial, projection, and blame
Strong need for look-good image
Win/lose mind-set
Attitude of entitlement
Self-absorbed
Short attention span

Affect

Empty and cold
Mock or faking of feelings when needed
Lack of remorse
Charming and slick
Depressed for a short time when caught
Angry intimidation

Interpersonal relationships

Wreckage following parasitic relationships
Shallow and self-serving
Strong need for control
Abusive and demanding

Patterns of substance abuse

If it feels good, do it twice
The more, the better
Polysubstance use

Adolescents with a coexisting borderline personality disorder

Presenting problems

Self-harm, self-mutilation
Suicide attempts; drug, alcohol overdoses
Angry attacks on others, unprovoked
Problems with authority

Thinking

Black-and-white
Numerous thinking errors
Devaluation
Preoccupation with pain and death
Negative world view
Get you before you get me
Help me! But you can't!

Affect

Self-loathing
Anger toward self and others
Extremely volatile
Depression

Interpersonal relationships

Hot/cold
Too intense, too quick
Love/hate
Enmeshment
Overidentification
Charming and seductive
Lack of consistent peer group

Patterns of substance abuse

Episodic substance abuse
Polysubstance use

Adolescents with a coexisting bipolar disorder

Presenting problems

Sexual promiscuity
Highly impulsive
Hyperactive
Legal problems

Affect

Elation/mania
Irrationality
Agitation
Depression/anger

(continued)

TABLE 9. (*continued*)

Runaway	Interpersonal relationships
Truancy	Strong need for social interactions
Angry outbursts	Brief
Thinking	Intense quality
Use of thinking errors	Quantity of relationships
Rapid thoughts	Seductive
Short attention span	Patterns of substance abuse
Easily distracted	Polysubstance use
Grandiose	
Delusional	

Adolescents with a coexisting schizophrenic disorder

Presenting problems	Affect
Psychosis	Flat, empty quality
Depression	Pacing, agitation
Suicide attempts	Depression, withdrawal
Bizarre behavior	Interpersonal relationships
Erratic violent behavior	Isolative
Thinking	Separate from group
Crazy, weird quality	Lack of peer group
Psychotic	Patterns of substance abuse
Concrete	Polysubstance use
Paranoid	

this story to adolescents when helping them to understand the concept of faith.

> Two men were sitting alone waiting for a bus. One of the men wore the collar of a Catholic priest. The other man turned to the priest and said, "I once prayed to your God to save my life and he failed me!" The priest smiled and said, "Tell me, my son, of your prayer." The man went on to tell how he had been lost in the Arctic cold of Alaska; he had no food or shelter and was certain he was going to die. In his last breath, he begged God to save him from death. The priest smiled and said, "But son, God did not fail you. You are alive." The man replied, "God didn't do anything. Some Eskimo showed me the way out."

We try to help the adolescent understand that the Higher Power works through people and that Eskimos are everywhere helping us when we most need help. We ask the youth to make lists of the Eskimos or people who have been helpful to him/her personally. We discuss these helpers in group counseling.

Step 3 requires the adolescent to turn his/her will and life over to the care of God as he/she understands Him. Counselors need to help the adolescent find an appropriate Higher Power. We discourage youth from choosing heavy metal rock music groups, doorknobs, or other unlikely sources of spiritual contact. Most often youth choose the AA group itself if they are uncomfortable with a more traditional view of God or have difficulty with the abstract concept of a Higher Power. Given that the United States is increasingly multicultural, understanding the spiritual beliefs of such groups as Hispanics or Southeast Asians can assist the counselor in helping the second-generation adolescents of immigrant/ refugee parents accept the beliefs of their parents or help them work through their rebellion against this and achieve their own resolution.

Other Treatment Considerations

We believe that effective adolescent treatment often initially requires a milieu that is guided and controlled by staff. The staff must establish and enforce prorecovery behavior and develop and promote positive peers. This is most easily done in a residential or inpatient program but can be done on an outpatient basis. We are willing to try outpatient treatment with a dually diagnosed adolescent at least willing to own up, who is not in immediate danger of harmful acts, and who has an intact positive support system.

A milieu is more likely to be positive if there is a stable or level system with immediate consequences for behavior, both positive and negative. In inpatient units this can be part of the program. Another useful strategy in residential programs is to reduce the privileges of upper-level adolescents if lower-level adolescents act out. This promotes an alliance between staff and the upper-level adolescents. A prorecovery milieu will also forbid the wearing of clothes or symbols that point to identification with antisocial drug-using groups. Wearing satanic tee shirts or sporting pink hairdos only serves to maintain a negative identity and blocks surrender and acceptance of the new identity as a recovering alcoholic or addict. Similarly, staff should forbid "war stories." As nearly as possible the milieu should encourage prosocial dress and behavior and provide a schedule of daily activities resembling the real world of the adolescent. This includes provision for school time, family time, and play. A key prorecovery behavior to promote in adolescents is the challenging of negative behavior and thinking errors engaged in by others. Besides harnessing the power of their peers, this exercise in critical thinking helps reduce the number of enablers who passively watch the good kids confront the bad kids.

Enforcing a prorecovery milieu in an outpatient program is more challenging, but it an be done. The level drops (access to privileges as an incentive to cooperate) of the home behavior contract discussed at greater length in the next chapter help to motivate the adolescents to adopt positive behavior. With conduct disordered adolescents, we have used such things as having private groups of "one" with special Step 1 assignments. This "image challenge," if done appropriately, can be a motivator. With borderline-type adolescents (generally female), membership in a same-sex group with a good milieu can take advantage of the strong pressure for conformity with the peers and of the bonding that quickly takes place. The group then has the power to influence behavior with threats of abandonment (suspension from the group and more individualized therapy) for failing to be sufficiently prorecovery.

We will often make a contingency plan with the adolescent and the family that if the youth fails in the outpatient setting then the youth will enter a more intensive setting. We view failure in the outpatient setting as a lesson in powerlessness and keeping a youth "on the waiting list" another form of corral. Requiring adolescents early in treatment to attend a designated 12-step group where a staff member is present to take attendance, monitor behavior, and coordinate with parents has proven to be a productive tactic.

Even more than with adults and especially on an outpatient basis, strong case management is essential for success with adolescents, especially those who evidence a conduct disorder. Frequent updates and sufficient communication among all parties who are part of the corral helps to defeat splitting (attempts to divide and conquer the adults), monitor behavior, and orchestrate responses. For example, we immediately phone the parent or legal guardian if the minor misses a session. Updates to schools occur at least monthly. If there is noncompliance or escalation of proscribed behavior, a staff meeting is useful for implementing last-chance agreements or at least getting everyone on the same page. This unscheduled crisis response is time-consuming but probably critical to the success of the program.

Working with the various systems of the adolescent is essential. Chapter 10 discusses family work in more detail. But sometimes returning the adolescent inpatient to the family is impossible. In cases where abuse is present or where the parents' alcoholism is so acute that the adolescent's recovery would be jeopardized if he/she were sent home, then alternative placement arrangements become essential. If sexual or physical abuse is identified during the course of treatment, we always report it to the appropriate authorities. We believe the secrecy of use must be broached if healing is to begin. We always put the safety of the child first. It would be wonderful if all adolescents had an Aunt Irene or a special relative who could provide an extended family resource to the child when immediate family members were not available. Halfway houses and group homes for adolescents, where staying clean and sober is a focus, are also extremely helpful in these cases. Sadly, in most cases, neither of these options is available. Underfunded public agencies have stretched their resources to the limit. If the adolescent is 16 or 17, early emancipation may be an option. In this case we assist the adolescent in completing his/her GED (graduate equivalency diploma), getting and keeping a job, and finding a place to live.

Where resources for placement outside the home are not available or the home situation is not so acutely dysfunctional, we do try to work with a parent or parents on problematic chemical use or subpar parenting styles. Less serious problems of this sort may be handled in the family session as part of the home behavior contract process. These sessions provide the opportunity to promote appropriate parenting and a safer environment. Agreements about a chemical-free home or no-hands-on (i.e., nonviolent) behavior contract are written down. Most of the time the parent or parents are able to comply with this, and we discuss noncompliance in follow-up sessions. Attendance at a parents' group reinforces these changes through the education and discussion that takes place there.

If problems continue or there are medium levels of such problems to start, we take a more gradual approach. As part of our family counseling we ask the parents to take psychological testing. We then meet separately with the parents to review the results of the "objective" testing and discuss any concerns we have. We use the procedures of motivational counseling to attempt to enhance the willingness of the parent or parents to do something about their own problems. This might involve getting an independent chemical dependency assessment or going for a medication evaluation for depression. We keep the adolescent out of these sessions in the belief that parents will be more forthright and feel less of a need to defend their authority by being "perfect" if the adolescent is not present. Moving the locus of the final assessment out of the family sessions has allowed us to continue to work with the family in some capacity if the family member rejects the assessor's findings or the assessment in some other way blows up.

We absolutely believe in the need for adolescents to have their own individual therapist while another counselor does the family therapy. Adolescents must feel free to be able to talk honestly and without fear of their parents knowing everything that is going on. Clear boundaries are imperative. This doesn't mean that parents are kept in the dark. Our family therapists are the contact points for parents to express concerns and to get summary overviews of progress. The exception to this is working with conduct-disordered adolescents. While we still use a set of two therapists, we encourage frequent contact among all parties to decrease the chances of being manipulated and split off from the "corral." Also, one of the biggest temptations in doing this kind of work with adolescents is to get quick points by joining with them in moaning about their parents. However, failure to ultimately challenge this stance keeps adolescents in the victim role and does not teach the self-responsibility that is part of recovery. Periodic updates between the two therapists will keep everyone apprised of "reality" and hopefully balanced in their views of the teen and the rest of the family.

For those too young to emancipate and who have no residential alternative, if our other attempts go nowhere, we try to focus the adolescent on achieving psychological emancipation despite unavoidable residence in the dysfunctional family home. We help the youngster understand the difference between his/her problem and his/her parents' problems. We encourage such youngsters to identify safe and supportive people and places—such as a friendly neighbor, an AA meeting, or the local church—that they can use for support and time-outs from their family. Occasionally this works, but often the youth relapses. We have often seen these youth become reinvolved with chemicals and even return to the streets. Their sobriety did not provide a roof over their head or food in their stomach, nor did it satisfy their safety and esteem needs.

Coordination with schools is extremely important. Besides providing excellent collateral data, the program staff and school personnel can work on developing remedial school programs designed to meet any special educational needs the adolescent may have. Many schools offer groups supporting sobriety and providing prorecovery peers. Schools can also monitor progress and detect a relapse. Probation officers, child protective service workers, and other involved service providers can serve similar functions. By having this group of people work together as a team and become involved in all phases of care, the chances of a successful outcome will increase. These other systems can also provide contingencies for enforcing treatment plans such as revocation of parole and return to a supervised living situation if the youth relapses.

Relapse Prevention

The dually diagnosed adolescent will benefit from all the strategies and services for preventing relapse outlined in the last few chapters in the sections for specific diagnoses. Particularly important is that he/she learn to have fun and resocialize with a clean and sober peer group.

Relapse rates for adolescents after leaving the structure of treatment are higher than for adults in our experience. However, all is not lost.

Our experience has been that adolescents that we have treated circle back around for additional treatment much earlier than they might have, had they never been treated. Treatment has inoculated them to some extent, and there remains a part of them that observes the progression of their addiction and says, "See, that's what they were talking about." This is particularly likely to happen with dually diagnosed adolescents without conduct disorders after they leave the home and find out that it wasn't all their parents' fault, after all.

THE ADOLESCENT SURVIVOR
OF CHILDHOOD TRAUMA
Key Clinical Issues

Dually disordered adolescents, like the dually disordered adults, present with numerous psychiatric issues and a variety of addiction problems as well. However, it has been our clinical experience that many of the dually diagnosed teens that we see suffer also from some degree of post-traumatic stress disorder and comorbid substance use disorders.

Trauma-based syndromes and substance use disorders are distressingly common in youth. The PTSD triad of symptoms includes (1) anxious arousal and avoidance, (2) intrusions, and (3) numbing (American Psychiatric Association, 1994). Trauma and addiction interact in alarming ways. There is high correlation between parents having a substance abuse disorder and the occurrence of physical and sexual abuse directed toward their children or partners (Meichenbaum, 1994). A history of childhood sexual and physical abuse increases the risk of developing a substance use disorder (Triffleman, Marmar, Delucchi, & Ronfeldt, 1995; Brown & Anderson, 1991).

Individuals suffering from a trauma-based disorder often have unique and heightened negative reactions to addictive chemicals. For example, the stimulants can often precipitate flashbacks and affective states associated with prior trauma, as can withdrawal symptoms (van der Kolk, 1994). Addictive chemicals (and at times even antidepressants) used originally to relieve dysphoric feelings will, with long-term use, actually exacerbate feelings of depression and anxiety (Kranzler & Liebowitz, 1988). A history of childhood trauma is associated with an increased risk of experiencing additional, later traumas, even independent of other risk factors (Boney-McCoy and Finkelhor, 1996; Breslau et al., 1995; Dutton et al., 1994). Abuse of chemicals increases the risk of exposure to traumas such as accidents as well as physical and sexual assaults, and prior substance abuse and dependence appear to increase the risk of developing a trauma-based syndrome in response to traumatic stress (Meichenbaum, 1994). For the adolescents, their exposure to violence is even greater due to drinking games of rapid intake and gang initiations involving violence.

Addicted teen survivors personify other treatment challenges because of additional characteristics these clients often present (Evans & Sullivan, 1995). These include the following:

1. *Denial.* Many survivors have well-developed denial systems that tend to operate in the present as well as the past. Denial has become an automatic response to any situation associated with anxiety for these individuals. Automatically "avoiding" awareness of their true feelings, needs, or options or avoiding situations needing attention is a set-up for impoverished and ineffective living because of the resulting confusion and indecision. This automatic and intense denial will also operate in regard to examining their drug use.

2. *Hypersensitivity.* A nearly universal characteristic of survivors is excessive emotional hypersensitivity and its related difficulties. This hyperawareness of the body language, moods, and the meaning "behind the words" is a highly functional defense mechanism. Add in adolescence and there is super hypersensitivity.

3. *Control struggles.* Strong needs for control are a fundamental issue for all adolescents and, coupled with survivors issues, this is indeed an issue that must be addressed clinically. Control refers to all the ways a person attempts to influence self and others to conform to a desired outcome through the exercise of willpower.

4. *Difficulties in trusting others.* Survivors almost always have difficulties with trust. Trust refers to a person's confidence that he/she can count on persons or events to be safe, reliable, or simply predictable. Just as survivors from a plane crash may no longer feel safe flying due to a perceived violation of trust, survivors from other types of trauma also have issues related to trust. The classic violation of trust occurs when parents are the abusers. Children expect that their parents are going to protect them and keep them safe. When this basic sense of safety is violated, tremendous damage is done. When abuse occurs inside the family, then there is neither safety nor support. The child feels both abused and abandoned. Children who experience this type of betrayal have experienced the most serious type of trust violation. This leaves the survivor with the strong impression that "important people cannot be trusted" (Briere & Runetz, 1988; Conte & Schuerman, 1987). Difficulties in trusting are typically generalized to various groups, people, or situations. In a sense survivors' distrust issues constitute a form of paranoia. Pervasive distrust limits the survivor's ability to ask for, and receive, help and support from others. This often leads to isolation and personal rigidity.

Unable to reach out for support, yet feeling overwhelmed and alone, the survivor is caught up in a self-defeating pattern of behavior.

5. *Distortions in the sense of responsibility.* Survivors wrestle with who is responsible for the abuse. Blaming themselves for the abuse is a common response of survivors. Many survivors will also have the experience of being blamed for the abuse by others when they first tell someone about the abuse. Their answer then generalizes to other life situations, leading to a distorted sense of overresponsibility. Many such children, as they head into their adolescence, then rebel very strongly in the opposite direction, as if to say "I've had enough." Extreme swings between over- and underresponsibility are common.

6. *Problems with anger.* Difficulties in expressing and reacting to anger are extremely common among teenaged addicted survivors. These difficulties take a number of forms. A common pattern that survivors show is an oscillation between rage and depression. Suppressing resentments alternates with temper outbursts. Typically the temper explosion is out of proportion to the situation at hand. Startled and frightened by their own level of rage, fearful of retaliation from others, or guilty about having displayed any feelings at all, the survivor swings back into being shut down.

7. *Unusual thinking and behavior.* Many survivors experience and demonstrate feelings, thoughts, and actions that are unusual. Unstable moods are common among survivors. Many survivors alternate between being shut down and flat, being full of rage, consumed by paralyzing fear, and tumbling into "black hole" depressions. Many survivors are constantly on an emotional roller-coaster. Sometimes seemingly minor events trigger this rush of feelings and at others times intense fear, anger, or other feelings come out of the blue with no obvious trigger. For the addicted adolescent survivor, mood swings are so commonplace that they end up being a central treatment concern for preventing relapse of both drug use and self-destructive behavior.

8. *Difficulty with spirituality.* Many survivors profess to be angry at God or feel that they are unworthy of God's love. These individuals have a difficult time with the spiritual components of 12-step programs and have difficulty with the conversion experience needed for change. The limited thinking range of the typical teen and shortcomings in abstract reasoning make the challenge of Steps 1–3 even more notable.

9. *Reenactment of self-defeating behavior.* A key concept for understanding trauma is the notion of reenactment (van der Kolk, 1989). Reenactment refers to the phenomenon of physiological and psychological repetition of the trauma—in both actual and symbolic ways—that survivors exhibit. Clients have an astounding ability to repeat problematic behav-

ior over and over, leading to increased damage and a sense of therapeutic pessimism.

10. *Alienation from others.* Teenagers are, of course, well known for their preoccupation with how well they fit in. Survivors' deeply ingrained sense of shame and inconsistent attachment lead to strong feelings of being detached and different from others and of not fitting in. Poor social skills are common. This contributes to the seduction of relationships based on getting high or loaded and of groups organized around anti-social activity.

Facilitating Change with Addicted Female Survivors

Our research outcomes and clinical work suggest that the internal pain caused by adolescents' trauma serves as an internal motivator to get "safe and sober." This motivator is the key factor leading to transformative change. External motivators are important, but safety and sobriety are the primary influences on clients' decision to change.

Courage is necessary for change to occur. The need for courage is typically activated by life problems so uncomfortable that change *must* occur. However, courage based purely on self-will has its limitations in the Twelve Step philosophy (Alcoholics Anonymous, 1976). Alcoholics Anonymous describes the process of this spiritual shifting and conversion experience as the bedrock of the recovery program.

AA taps into an ancient wisdom as the source of spiritual awareness, making available to its members the long and rich tradition of the spirituality of imperfection. The spirituality of imperfection begins by recognizing that trying to be perfect is the most tragic of human flaws. AA suggests, "First of all, we had to quit playing God." According to the way of life that flows from this insight, it is only by stopping all attempts to play God—by accepting the inability to control every aspect of life, including alcohol—that peace and serenity can be found (Alcoholics Anonymous, 1976).

Spiritual thinkers have always distinguished between those who have claimed to have changed and those who are open to change (Kurtz & Ketchum, 1996). A distinction underlying all change is the notion of a "conversion" experience. The founders of Alcoholics Anonymous were cautious of using this term, as it had too many religious connotations. Instead, AA members prefer the term "spiritual awakening" (Alcoholics Anonymous, 1957).

The essential lesson demonstrating this spiritual awakening is demonstrated in the meetings of Alcoholics Anonymous. At AA meetings, this spiritual awakening or conversion experience is detailed through the members' telling of their unique individual stories. The recommended way to tell a recovery story is to first discuss "what it was like" (when drinking or using), "what happened" and "what it is like now" (to cement one's own conversion experience and help galvanize others') (Alcoholics Anonymous, 1957).

The story below will illustrate this process. "Jane" told her story in the interviews that were part of Dr. Katie Evans's dissertation research exploring the conversion experience in teenaged females who are addicted survivors of trauma (Evans, 1999). A case overview is first, followed by the client's own story, which also includes comments by Dr. Evans.

A COMPOSITE CASE EXAMPLE: "JANE"

Jane's mother worked as a nurse. It was through her working in a local hospital that Jane's mother met the man who would be Jane's father, a doctor. Jane's mother and father fell deeply in love. They had been together only 3 months when Jane's mother got pregnant. For the first 3 years of her life Jane enjoyed both a father and mother who adored her. Jane was always a very sensitive person. From the time that she was born, her parents marveled at her contemplative style—unusual, they thought, for a baby.

Then, as if overnight, Jane's father moved out, leaving Jane and her mother to fend for themselves. He did, however, initially keep in contact with Jane and her mother, but over time, they saw him less and less frequently and eventually no longer had contact with him. Financial struggles and day care problems led Jane's mother to work double shifts. Jane often slept over at the babysitter's house due to her mother's long work hours. Jane's previous adoration and attentive upbringing came to a sudden crash. This sudden uprooting of Jane and being forced into a new home environment with a "new room" left Jane feeling quite confused and frightened. She, like most young children struggling with narcissistic issues, assumed that her mother had gone away because she was a bad girl. Jane tried harder and harder to "be perfect," but her mother continued to be away. Jane developed nightmares, which often played out as night terrors. No one could comfort the frightened child as she cried in the middle of the night "please don't leave me!" The loss of her father, who had suddenly left, complicated by her sense of loss of her mother due to her return to work, left Jane with anxiety symptoms related to abandonment.

The loss that Jane experienced, which affected her sense of safety and security, became even more of an active traumatic event due to the effects of the babysitter. At a developmental stage where Jane should be separating and seeing herself more as an individual, with the comfort of a secure attachment that mother was there, Jane experienced just the opposite. She began to see the world as unsafe and one where she only had herself to count on to survive. Jane recalls being very afraid at night to go to sleep. To complicate matters, the babysitter's fundamentalist religious beliefs played out in warnings to Jane about "God knows everything you think; do you want to burn in hell or go back with Jesus if he comes to get you tonight?" These bedtime warnings only increased the nightmares, and fear-based thinking. Jane grew to think of God as a source of fear, not a source of love, faith, and trust. God became another critical authority figure, which Jane now had to please or burn in hell. To add to this challenge, Jane attended church with her babysitter, where Jane recalls hearing the preacher saying that "Jesus is always watching you, even when you are asleep." The preacher also was quite focused on what would happen at Armageddon: the notion was that only those who "lived in Christ's path, completely" would make it to heaven. Those who sinned or who had not been "saved" would go to hell. Jane recalls lying in her bed at night frightened that God would come, and she and her mother would not be taken to heaven. This nightly torment was Jane's belief that the house of the babysitter was haunted—haunted by Jesus, God, angels, and ghosts. Jane reports a number of incidents where she heard the moving of "spirits" in the house. The babysitter also believed in these spirits and would take Jane with her as she prayed in different rooms asking that "God would dispel the evil spirits from the home."

As Jane grew older, she became more independent from the babysitter. Jane made new friends that were not members of the church. Jane, terrified to be attached and yet afraid to be alone, used her adolescent separation as a way to remove herself from the babysitter's rules, home, and life. These new friends were "more fun." Her new peers enjoyed drinking and smoking marijuana. Jane had never experienced what had been called "sin" or the "dark side of life." Jane's choices led the babysitter to call Jane a "condemned person" and insist that "this sinner" was removed from her care. Jane's emerging adolescence, coupled with her new friends and angry new attitudes, led the babysitter to "ban her from her home, as she was dancing with the Devil." Jane was devastated by the rejection by the babysitter.

Jane never considered what part her drug and alcohol use was playing in her metamorphosis from angel to delinquent. Jane stayed home with her mother and was left unsupervised a good deal of the time due to the mother's work schedule. Jane's mother became aware that her daughter was drinking and was very concerned, yet felt helpless to intervene. Jane's mother had told her that she best be careful with alcohol as there were many alcoholics in her family tree. In spite of these warnings, Jane found that alcohol offered her something which she had never experienced before. It made the pain stop. Jane began to get into trouble at home and school. Her old church friends did not want anything to do with Jane. Feeling abandoned and alone Jane acted out her hurt and fears by an increased isolation from adults. Jane's sense that she had somehow "sinned," caused a blow to her developing sense of self and added to already built-up feelings of hopelessness and depression. Jane began to stay at home alone at night while her mother worked. Alone at night, Jane began to drink. Alcohol seemed to fill the vacuum in her life and numb the pain. At first Jane would have only one or two drinks, but then, as her tolerance increased, so did her belief that alcohol was the only way to numb the pain.

Jane's introversion grew along with her sense of isolation. Jane required alcohol to be with people, especially men. Jane had begun to experience blackouts and memory loss when drinking. One evening after too much to drink Jane met a "cute and wonderful guy." Due to her extreme inebriation, Jane's friends took her home, but not before she had gotten the phone number of the boy who had sparked her interest. With Jane tucked safely in bed her friends bade her "good night." Jane could not get the boy out of her mind. Then Jane remembered, "I have his phone number!" Jane called the number and the boy answered. Shocked that he was home so early, all that she could think to say was "come over now, no one is home but me." Jane fell asleep; she was awakened by the presence of someone lying beside her. "Who is there?" Jane asked through slurred speech. "It's me. I am here to keep you company," the boy said. Then he gradually began to undress her. Jane's sleepful state made the removal of her clothes an easy task. As the boy climbed on top of her and began to enter her, Jane awoke. "What? Who are you? I am still a virgin, don't, please . . ." The boy responded that it was "too late now," and "besides, I am going to make you my girlfriend." For the next year and a half Jane dated Trent. The "dating" involved Trent coming over after Jane had drunk enough to "feel social" and, of course, during the time Jane's mother was at work. Jane decided that he must really "love her" to spend so much time with her.

The relationship became more problematic as Trent became overly controlling of everything that Jane did. He didn't like her friends or for her to wear certain clothes. When Jane tried to be assertive, Trent started abusing her physically. First it was a grab or a shove, then it was a slap, then finally came a time when, in a heated argument, Trent blackened both of Jane's eyes and hurt her arm. Jane threatened to break up with him. Trent said, "Don't bother, you're just an alcoholic slut anyway!" Devastated by the breakup, Jane began to cut on herself to punish herself for being bad. Then one night, overwhelmed with feelings of loss and abandonment, Jane tried to kill herself by taking an overdose of her mother's sleeping pills with a bottle of vodka. Jane's mother came home early from work, found the vodka bottle and the empty sleeping pill bottle, and rushed Jane to the hospital. After a week in intensive care, Jane was able to return home. It was then that both Jane and her mother knew she needed help.

Jane began her story with deep thought and a quiet voice. "I don't know when or how I first started drinking. I can't remember the first time I drank, because I just think about why I drank. There were so many things that I had to think about and I didn't want to think about them, I didn't want to face life, sort of. I mean, I had a lot of low points: a lot of things that people would say, 'That is depressing, really depressing.' But I kind of realized that and I knew that I didn't want the rest of my life to be like that." Jane was asked about her internal pain and how drinking interfaced with that pain. Commenting further about her drinking, Jane reported, "Mostly I drank alone, I had a secret life. I drank a little in social situations, but somehow I was able to control that. But I would go home and get drunk alone, to try not to feel anything. Bad things happened when I drank socially, so I found it safer to drink alone."

Jane told her story of growing up as follows: "My mom and dad were never married; they lived together for probably 3 years. At the time we were living as a family my father was still married to someone else. He had separated from his wife to come and live with us. I don't remember much about him while we were living with him, but I never loved him or never really cared that much about him. He was never an important person in my life and he never will be. He was just kind of there, and I haven't seen him for probably 2 to 3 years now. I never think about him and I never miss him."

In response to a question of "What was your contact like when he moved out from you and your mother?", Jane responded, "It was very frequent at first, very frequent, but as I grew up it became more infrequent and more sporadic. I think he realized that I had no feelings for him, although I never did tell him or say that. I wasn't expected to, my mom said that he understood. I just had no desire to see him, and I don't think that he had any desire to see me, knowing that I had no feelings for him. The visits became less frequent, until finally they stopped." As Jane discussed her rejection of her father's love she did so with such a vehemence that it raised the question of who she was trying to convince that she never loved him. It was reminiscent of the young child who states, "If you don't play with me, then I won't be your friend!" Jane held herself responsible for her father leaving because she "never loved him and had no desire to see him." Therefore she concluded that "I don't think that he had any desire to see me, knowing that I had no feelings for him."

Jane went on to describe the aftermath of her father's leaving. "He never divorced his wife, so when he left he went back to her. Then they had their own child, a son. I think that he is 8 years younger than I am. His name is Alex. We never met him. I have seen pictures. The kid looks exactly like me. I think that someday I would like to meet him, but not while he is still a child." Jane's motivation to meet her half-brother as an adult had been processed in early sessions of therapy. It was Jane's wish "not to upset him—he is just a kid." Thus once again she is sacrificing her own needs and desires to try to give to another child that which was not given to her, and this is another survivor response. This ability to empathize and protect others while abandoning self is another aspect of posttraumatic stress disorder.

Jane described that, after her father left, "my mother began to work nights as a night-shift nurse up at the medical school. More recently I enjoyed the fact that she worked nights, as I had a lot of unsupervised time. This gave me an opportunity to drink alone whenever I wanted. When I was younger, I needed a place to sleep at nights. My mom found a lady where I had my own room, and she provided me sort of a second home. I felt like the other people which lived there were also like my family. The woman Joyce was sort of a mother and grandmother all rolled up into one. But she was a very religious person, and I was kind of forced into religion—I really didn't have a choice. I started staying there when I was about 3 years old, right after my dad had left." Jane explained that this was her first introduction to religion. "It was all very frightening, I mean she was a born-again Christian and it was, you know, if you aren't born again, and you get to the end, when Jesus comes down you won't be saved and taken to heaven with Him, you will burn in the fires of hell forever! You know, Christ just coming down any moment and I am not going to be one of the ones that goes up, made me feel frightened, angry, and somehow abandoned all at the same time." This hypervigilant response to her surroundings and fear that she will be left are classic symptoms of posttraumatic stress disorder.

Asked if she experienced any bad dreams or nightmares, Jane responded, "No. For a long time when I was there I didn't dream at all; which is odd, because I remember dreams when I was 3 or 4 years old, but I don't remember much about those early dreams. Then the bad dreams started. It sounds kind of odd, but the house had a lot of really odd things that would go wrong with it, just really bizarre, you know, cabinets opening." This writer commented that it sounded as if she thought the house was haunted. Jane replied, "Yeah, it kind of sounds weird." This writer asked if living there felt unsafe and scary? Jane continued, "Yeah, the house alarm would just go off in the middle of the night all by itself. They didn't have any pets inside, and they had had people come out and check the alarm, but it kept going off. Oh, man, it was scary! I remember just being in bed and always trying to look like the bed was empty, like always having the covers over my face, trying to make the bed look like it was sort of just messed up instead of an actual person being there. Just in case something happened, maybe they would overlook me. But, for a long time I couldn't sleep." Jane describes bad dreams and fear-based dissociation, which are both common trauma-based responses.

Jane continued, "Then later on there were the boyfriend problems—you know, the sex stuff. Do I have to talk about that here? I don't want to on tape." Sensing Jane's lack of safety in sharing these more intimate details of her trauma, this writer responded, "No, not if you are uncomfortable sharing that particular abuse on tape." Developing and maintaining a sense of safety and avoiding any trauma reenactment during the therapeutic process are keys to effective survivor counseling.

Jane thought carefully when questioned about what motivated her to get clean and sober. "Well, I think that before I came here I wanted to be sober. I think that coming here gave me the strength to do it, kind of like the tools. I don't think that anyone really pushed me into being sober. I think that they gave me the option and told me, 'Hey, look at what is going to happen to you if you don't,' so I think that I took the things that others said to me to heart, and I just made myself stop drinking and get help."

Jane felt that the initial motivation for starting treatment was generated externally. Her mother was the catalyst for getting her into counseling in the first place. Yet, Jane also thought that during the course of treatment she stopped doing treatment for her mother and developed positive transference toward the therapist. Through this positive transference the therapist served as a transitional "Higher Power" until the subjects had made peace with their childhood God and developed their own personal relationship, a conversion experience.

Through working the 12-step program as part of the integrated treatment approach, Jane said that she had "fired" her old authoritative God and had developed a personal relationship with a benevolent loving God. The transference between the subjects and the clinician served as a transitional model for an unconditional love experience from an authoritative source. This was the needed bridge for the subjects' own personal conversion experience and their desired change based on internal motivation.

The integration of spirituality, psychology, mental health concepts, and recovery notions are the combination we find that produces successful outcomes. Jane participated in weekly individual counseling with Dr. Evans as well as a group therapy for addicted teenaged female survivors that met weekly. Jane had family counseling. We required Jane to attend two 12-step meetings weekly. The majority of our adolescent survivors do well and have good outcomes with this treatment approach.

CHAPTER 10

Working with Families

A codependent is someone who, when she is drowning,
someone else's life flashes before her eyes.
—ANONYMOUS

Clinical attention to the families of dually diagnosed clients is crucial for a variety of reasons. Families are a source of accurate information on clients' status and also a source of motivation for initiating change. Responses of the family members to psychiatric and chemical use problems can either aid or interfere with dual recovery. Family members also deserve attention because of the enormous distress and difficulties that persons suffering from dual disorders can cause. In this chapter we discuss some of the issues facing the service provider working with the families of dually diagnosed clients and present some approaches for working with these families.

THE ROLE OF THE FAMILY

Families are a key factor in the causes and conditions associated with substance abuse and psychiatric disorders. One mode of causality is through genetic and developmental means. Children of alcoholics (COAs), for example, are themselves at increased risk of substance use disorders, conduct disorders, and cognitive deficits of various kinds, as well as being subject to greater physical and sexual abuse (Gotham & Sher, 1996; Chassin, Curran, Hussong, & Colder, 1996). Family members can also make either a negative contribution toward the maintenance and exacerbation of the client's problems or become a key to the solution. Alcohol use can increase the negativity of both partners in marital interactions, and families with a drinking alcoholic member are rigid in their functioning (Leonard & Roberts, 1998; Steinglass, 1981). High levels of expressed emotion (EE) by family members increase the rates of relapse for schizophrenia, mood disorders, and substance use disorders (O'Farrell et al., 1998). Marital distress can be an important contributor to major depression (Beach & O'Leary, 1992). On the other hand, family members can help the clinician serve as a monitor of clients' true status (Galanter, 1993). A comprehensive review of the research on couple and family interventions concluded that involvement of spouses and other family members enhances treatment outcomes for alcohol dependence, schizophrenia, and major depression, decreasing the number of such things as dropping out from treatment and relapses (Baucom et al., 1998).

Family members themselves also benefit from treatment. Treatment of drug and alcohol problems decreases family crises and difficulties (e.g., Gibson, Sorenson, Wermuth, & Bernal, 1992).

FAMILY THERAPY APPROACHES
The Systems Model

Three family models form the basis for interactions in the alcohol and drug treatment field (Margolis & Zweben, 1998), the first of which is the systems model.

Family Rules

The systems approach attempts to make explicit the implicit predictable patterns, or "rules," operating in the family, such as "Don't upset Mommy, she's weak and needs protection" or "Only Daddy's needs count." Black, an early writer in the field, identified the "Don't talk, feel or trust" rules (Black, 1991).

Myths unique to each family constitute another set of "rules." Most families have stories or myths that they pass on to the next generation. Attitudes toward life are often shaped by these family beliefs. Some of these beliefs may be very helpful—such as those stories, for example, that promote honesty or hard work. Other times these family myths are very destructive. Take, for example, the family that grows up with little money and is always worried whether there will be enough to "make ends meet." The belief that there is never enough can be passed on to the next generation, causing frugal hoarding and exaggerated economic insecurity. This might be so extreme that it results in problems within the family or in the workplace. Other members of the next generation might tend toward the opposite extreme, in counterreaction. Feeling that money only incites money grubbing and vowing not to be like their parents, the offspring can become shopaholics and throw money away in order to play the big shot. In both situations the family's preoccupation with not having enough leads to scarcity-oriented thinking in generations that follow.

Family therapists will find it helpful to come to know a family's myths. Inquiring about family stories can thus yield considerable insight, as the underlying beliefs may be governing various undercurrents within the family.

We have observed several informal "rules" that may actually interfere with initiating change through the families' own efforts or through treatment. The first of these is that the family cannot do anything differently until blame has been fully and appropriately allocated. This results in the "blame" game, in which family members alternate between anger ("you're to blame") and shame ("I'm to blame") and expend all their energy in debating and trying to resolve this issue. A variant of this is the "why" question, an especially good one for intellectualizers. Family members get caught up in being right rather than being happy or effective. With this rule there is a tendency to take the client's behavior as deliberately directed toward each family member. The collective wounds of all the family members can produce a narcissistic nightmare at home and in the therapy room.

Another familiar but untrue rule is that "nothing will work—we've already tried everything." In this scenario, family members confuse powerlessness over another family member with helplessness to change their own behavior. This learned helplessness perpetrates a depressive stance of inaction and immobility. A third rule is that we can have a life only when the presenting problem is fixed. This pattern represents a mix of misplaced loyalty, vigilance directed toward potential threats and inappropriate fears that all is lost unless everything is fixed right now. "If I just say or do exactly the right thing, everything will be fine" is a fourth rule. This rule assumes that there is a right thing and that one person can control the other person's illness, both of which are untrue. A fifth false rule is that, once the person's symptoms subside, everything else will be OK. Recovery is a process and not an event, and the client's symptoms are not the cause of each and every problem in the family.

These rules are typically entrenched and potent, and they have the quality of hypnotic trances. Careful observation of family members who exhibit these patterns can be used to rebut their narrowed, fixated attention and the illogical logic of family-induced trance states.

Therapy must challenge these rules (or trances) if change is to occur. This requires therapists to intervene actively and decisively to disrupt entrenched patterns and to avoid getting "hypnotized" themselves. Interventions can include directives ("Stop it and everyone take a deep breath and look at me"), provision of information ("A lot of this is genetic, you know"), humor ("You can argue like that for free and on your own time; let's do something different in this office") and shock ("Let's just hope no one dies while we debate the latest theories on the causes of these problems"). Simply and directly commenting on the rules is a useful intervention as well. The goal is to promote a hopeful, helpful, remedy-oriented context for change—"to live in the solution, not the problem," as the AA slogan puts it.

Figure 2, created by Katie Evans and our former colleague J. Douglas Myers, summarizes some of these issues and strategies for intervening with families of dually disordered adolescents. We use the figure as a handout when training clinicians in the area of family myths.

Family Roles

The systems approach also attempts to educate family members about the roles in the family that have developed and that perpetuate the problem. Traditionally six roles are identified (Thombs, 1999). First and of course foremost is the *chemically dependent person.* Next is the *chief enabler,* usually the spouse, who protects the chemically dependent one from the consequences of his or her actions. Well-meaning and often facing constraints such as battering or financial dependence, the chief enabler attempts to keep things rolling along. The *family hero* is the child who outperforms at school and home and operates as a surrogate adult in the family. The hero child excels in both traditional achievements and also in taking care of others, thereby serving as the chief enabler's ally. However, the hero is not particularly good at taking care of his/her own needs and often ends up enabling others in their own relationships. The *scapegoat* is the child who acts out and becomes the focus of blame for the family's problems. Family members organize around repairing or reforming the scapegoat and thereby avoid tackling the other problems in the family. The scapegoat also makes a good candidate for this role because typically he/she has his/her own independent problems. The *lost child* "disappears" and placates others and avoids all conflict. Also, sometimes there is a *mascot,* a child who acts the clown and helps divert the family from the real problems. The goal of intervention is to help family members shift out of these roles through education and discussion of these roles and the development of more helpful ones. We do this through didactic presentations and discussions of material.

Boundaries and Functioning

Finally, the systems approach looks for inappropriately close (enmeshed) or distant (disengaged) boundaries and overly rigid or chaotic functioning, as well as inappropriate alliances across generations and out-of-

FIGURE 2. Family therapy with dually disordered youth (Katie Evans, PhD, NCACII, & J. Douglas Myers, PhD).

PHILOSOPHY

1. Dually disordered youth lack internal controls. External controls are needed.

2. Many families foster dependency by giving love, material objects, and support when the youth is in trouble and yet criticize the same person when he/she is *trying* to do well.

3. Often parents end up parenting by crisis. This leads to reactive parenting, not active parenting.

4. Reactive parenting is based on emotion, not logic. Consequencing is based on how angry, frightened, or hurt a parent is feeling at the time he/she determines the consequences or lack thereof; at a deeper level family members are reenacting their own unresolved painful story of growing up in a chaotic or disengaged family system. Adults take the myths (trance logic) of their own families and bring them to their new family and reenact the old patterns of feelings and behaviors.

5. These old myths (trances) that adults bring to the parenting relationship set the tone for the re-creation of the old fear-based reactive parenting styles that they learned in childhood.

6. Fear-based parenting leads to the absence of adults in the system. The adult "parent" is operating from a child's world view, which is fear-based. The wounds and mind-set of the parent are taught to the children. "Do as I say, not as I do" is the taproot of the family's double-bind logic.

7. Myths brought into a family through reactive parenting lead to a corruption of the system's ability to foster individualization and autonomy in the children who are being raised in this system. Fear-based or shame-based beliefs (trance logic) instill a stronger message than the hopeful words stated by the parent.
   Examples: of shame-based belief include
   "Yes, I see you got a B in English on your report card; that is really good, honey, but, how are you going to raise that B to an A?"
   "I guess with your grades you will have to marry well; and you probably won't get into college."
   "What's wrong now? You are just too sensitive."

8. Reactive parenting creates an emotionally volatile climate. In this "What's wrong now?" problem-focused system, the child is not taught how to manage feelings or behavior, or how to develop the necessary tools for a faith-based life.

THE REACTIVE PARENTING SYSTEM

Remember the 4 C's: Chaotic, Critical, Controlling, and Crisis-focused.

Myths (trance logic)

"Don't try or you will fail."
"Don't trust people outside the family."
"Don't get angry: feelings are bad, a problem to deal with."
"Do as I say, not as I do."
"You will probably fail, so why try?"
"Don't question [the myths] or you are bad."
"You won't be loved unless you do what I say and do."
"Be right, be perfect, don't ever make mistakes."

(continued)

FIGURE 2. (*continued*)

THE ACTIVE PARENTING SYSTEM

Incorporation of the 5 *S*'s: Safety, Structure, Skills, Serenity, Solution-based thinking.

Comment on family myths in therapy sessions

"Mr. Smith, I heard you say that Bob will fail without an education. Fail what?
"It sounds as if you doubt that life is full of choices; is there only one right road? Do you think that being right is more important than being happy?"

Write personal and family myths stories

Give assignments to write family myths and beliefs down and discuss them one-on-one or as a group.
Rewrite as a new faith-based story: "That Was Then, This Is Now."
Demonstrate the differences between the negative myth versus solution-based thinking.

Offer more helpful myths

"There are no mistakes, just lessons."
"Things turn out the way they are supposed to."
"Nothing happens in God's world by mistake."
"Visualize and actualize."
"You can be anything you choose to be."
"You don't need to be perfect to be perfectly happy."
"I would rather be happy than right."
"Ask for help. There are no stupid questions."
"Make mistakes so that, through learning what doesn't work, you can see what does."
"We have nothing to fear but fear itself."
"There is a bit of good in the worst of us and a bit of bad in the best of us."
"There is no Right or Wrong, only choices. Some are helpful choices, some are less helpful."
"You already have the answers. You just need to look where you have hidden them."

Faith-based over fear-based thinking: abundance versus scarcity

Model this during therapy sessions while also making process comments:
"We are here to discuss solutions to situations that used to be troubling."
"We have discussed what behavior and reactions were not helpful. Now let's discuss some ideas that may prove more helpful."
"There are lots of possible solutions. Let's discuss some and see if any might be helpful to you."

Structure the family situation with a home behavior contract

The contract offers logic, consistency, and predictability.

Teach affective containment and structure the sessions for safety

Use fair-fighting rules: no name calling, interrupting, or sarcasm.
Employ compliment sandwiches (compliment/concern/compliment).
Take breaks, provide containment for affect, and use breathing exercises and other trance-busting techniques.

Model an affirming and directive style (a model for parents)

Say "I like that" and "I wonder if . . ." rather than "That is good, *but* . . ."

Growing autonomy in all family members is achieved through faith-based win–win thinking: no right or wrong, just helpful or less helpful choices.

balance power differentials, and seeks to realign and rebalance them (e.g., Sells, 1998).

One common out-of-alignment boundary is the emotionally too close relationship that often develops between the oldest child and the non-drinking spouse. Over the years the oldest child becomes the confidant(e) and friend of that adult and operates as a pseudoadult. Interestingly, we have repeatedly observed a pattern wherein this child (the hero) suddenly (during adolescence) explodes into rage at the "weak" nonusing spouse and segues into the acting-out "bad child" (scapegoat).

A related pattern is the daughter who thinks her mother is too weak to stand up to the father or stepfather and takes on this battle through acting out. The daughter also both loves and resents the mother, the relationship being very ambivalent. One intervention for this is to ensure that the parent gets independent support and to give permission to the child to have his/her own life.

Another boundary conflict that we often see is a polarized parental coalition in which the stepparent is overly strict and the biological parent too permissive. This paralysis in parental functioning facilitates acting out by the adolescent and also degrades the marital relationship. An intervention that we use that is sometimes successful is to put the biological parent in charge of all discipline and give the stepparent permission to be "just a friend" to the adolescent and to support the biological parent after that person expresses support for the incredibly difficult, if not impossible, task that the stepparent has taken on (in being "just a friend"). Often the biological parent moves toward the "middle" as he/she is no longer distracted by the need to protect the child, and the child's negative behavior now becomes the focal point of annoyance.

Another problem we sometimes see is the single parent who inconsistently implements rules and consequences. Often there is a cycle of being too lax (because of fatigue, fear, neediness, and so forth) and then, with a buildup of frustration and resentment, of being too picky and stern. The home behavior contract described below is an excellent tool for increasing consistency and balance. In both marriage and family work, helping the chief enabler to "get out of the way of the crisis" is an important strategy. Once again, helping the chief enabler see that he/she could be more helpful by helping him/herself is crucial and often is accomplished by providing other sources of support, both emotional and material.

The Behavioral Model

The family behavioral model posits that skill deficits and inappropriate reinforcement of using behavior maintain and perpetuate the problem. For example, nagging the alcoholic about his/her drinking is a common response of the spouse attempting to influence the drinking partner. However, nagging may inadvertently accelerate the drinking through such mechanisms as escalating the power struggle, increasing negative affect, or giving the alcoholic rationalizations for further drinking. Another dysfunctional pattern that we have seen is that chemicals often provided the stimulus context for socializing, recreating, and having sex. With the chemicals absent, couples have to learn alternative ways to accomplish these functions.

Helping family members to use positive reinforcement of sober behaviors and put drinking behaviors in extinction can change the patterns in the marriage to more productive ones and result in increased participation in treatment of those with substance use disorders (e.g., Miller, Meyers, & Tonigan, 1999; Yoshioka, Thomas, & Ager, 1992). Contracting for abstinence, teaching problem-solving and communication skills, and implementing increased exchanges of positive behaviors between relationship partners are other interventions from within this model that supplement the client's individual treatment (O'Farrell, 1993). In marital therapy, for example, having spouses reactivate former idealizations can take place through encouraging realistic compliments. Doing something for the other that one knows the other spouse would appreciate and that one has freely picked to do starts to regenerate a positive atmosphere and pleasant reengagement. Frank discussions of fears of relapse and an action plan are also helpful in reducing some of the codependent enmeshment.

The Family Disease Model

The final influential model is the family disease model. Within this model, family members suffer from the "disease" of codependence. Beattie (1987) most successfully articulated and popularized the concept of codependence. Just as the addict or alcoholic has developed a distorted relationship with substances, the codependent has developed a distorted relationship with the chemically dependent individual. Codependents unsuccessfully attempt to control the addict, develop tolerance for deviant behavior, are preoccupied with the addict, give up important relationships and activities because of the addict, and so forth. It's as if the codependent is effectively addicted to the alcoholic.

Working a recovery program with the goal of detaching with love is the recommended remedy. Such a program entails attending Al-Anon meetings, working the steps, including Step 1 (admitting powerlessness over the addict), and getting a sponsor. It might also entail "abstaining" from relationships with someone who is practicing their addiction. Relapses can occur, and relapse prevention activities are appropriate.

"Didn't cause it, can't cure it, can't control it" is an Al-Anon slogan that can go a long way toward relieving spouses or parents of unrealistic guilt and shame. Presentations on these concepts and referral to Al-Anon can encourage family members to get into their own recovery. Explaining how this can help the client's recovery can take advantage of lingering codependent-based motivation to move family members into their own recovery.

THE THREE MODELS AND MENTAL HEALTH PROBLEMS

These three general models of family therapy approaches in the field of alcohol and drug treatment—namely, the systems model, behavioral model, and family disease model—also underlie interventions with mental health problems. In this field, three distinct approaches are specifically informed by concerns about particular mental health problems. Interpersonal psychotherapy (IPT) is an effective treatment. It views major depression as a potentially chronic disease and social role transitions and conflicts as key triggers for the onset of this disease (DeRubeis & Crits-Christoph, 1998). Therapy involves encouraging clients to let go of shame about their depression and to accept the role of a sick person while, at the same time, identifying the core role impasse and engaging in detailed specific problem-solving efforts. With this model in mind, we are careful to ask clients about how things are going at work and at home. This often elicits stressors in the form of marital difficulties and changes in jobs that appear to have precipitated a depression or other mental health problem.

The notion of expressed emotion (EE) was originally developed in the context of the family treatment of schizophrenia but has been extended to other disorders (O'Farrell et al., 1998). Persons suffering from schizophrenia and other disorders are very vulnerable to stress, and a major source of stress is the highly critical or demanding and intrusive relationship styles of relatives. Most interventions within this tradition use education, enhanced but detached monitoring of the client's status, problem solving, and encouragement of realistic expectations with families. At least for families with a member suffering from schizophrenia, long-term involvement with families and avoidance of emotionally charged family therapies seems to be important for success (Baucom et al., 1998). For example, we work with spouses to monitor compliance with medication and the general level of symptoms. We then have them call us to discuss any concerns and to schedule an appointment for their family member to come in. We also encourage them not to confront or challenge the client. Routine, periodic check-in meetings also help to avert crises. In some cases we have encouraged clients simply to avoid high-stress relatives who inevitably provoke an exacerbation of symptoms.

Developed by behavioral clinicians primarily focused on delinquent children, interventions that teach parents to implement consistent and appropriate consequences and be appropriately assertive in setting limits can substantially decrease adolescent acting out (Barkley, Edwards, & Robin, 1999). Our adolescent treatment program includes both a parent education component and family counseling that focuses on structuring the expectations and consequences for chemical use and other behavior through written contracts. We also focus on enhancing the parents' abilities to implement and maintain the structure despite the teens' inevitable attempts at countercontrol.

TREATMENT APPROACHES FOR DUAL RECOVERY

Consistent with our general strategy of seeing similarities and blending approaches from addiction and mental health treatments, we use family interventions with dually diagnosed clients as well.

Just as with the client, early and late recovery have different goals. Early recovery has the goal of family stability, where the emphasis is on a happy medium between chaos and rigidity and the setting of appropriate boundaries to avoid the extremes of enmeshment and disengagement. Later in recovery the emphasis within the family is more on growth and the enhancement of family members' relationships with one another. In our experience, the "outside-in" approach described in Chapter 2 also applies to families. Family work that leaps into in-depth emotional processing early on is bound to fail. First things first with families as well as the identified client. We provide safety and structure and skills prior to exploring painful feelings.

We have found the following approaches useful in early recovery. If the client is still unstable during the early-recovery stage of treatment, we prefer to work with family members and the client separately. The client has his/her own work to do, and family members need to feel safe to change without the fear of confrontation and a temper outburst from the client while doing their work.

Assessment

We require a parent or responsible adult to be present for assessments of adolescents. Apart from such issues as consent and payment, parents and others are important sources of information that is likely to be more accurate. Their contributions can also help to motivate the client in a positive direction. Even with adults, we strongly recommend that a significant other meet with us at the initial intake or the second session at the latest. We view any attempts by clients to deny releases of information or to prohibit such contacts as an indicator that they are either protecting their access to chemicals or protecting themselves from abuse, or both. This becomes a subject for immediate discussion and problem solving. Our own experience is that involvement by family members generally results in better outcomes and is worth the extra effort.

At the initial session or soon after, the opportunity is ripe to begin to shift the views of family members. This can occur through explaining the diagnoses, their causes and consequences, and the treatment plan. Psychological testing serves to make the process more detached and gives the provider more credibility. Getting everyone committed to the treatment plan is crucial. This is also the point at which providers and family members make decisions about the intensity of treatment required and, in some cases, the bottom lines that they will draw. Coordinating the corral through contact with employers, schools, parole and probation officers, and so forth is also a part of this initial treatment planning stage. Finally, joining with all involved members to formulate goals within the shared framework presents other opportunities to enhance motivation.

This is also a time when we sometimes switch to defining the significant other as the client. For example, we sometimes see spouses drag in their partners for "marital problems." These spouses then announce during the first session that the real problem is alcohol. Typically, the (presumed) addict then blows up and accuses the spouse of lying, being controlling, exaggerating, and so forth. Of course, this is both true and a diversion. Attempts to assess the alcohol issue are generally futile, and the addict may then storm out or refuse to schedule a follow-up visit. Sometimes the addict is open to treatment, especially after a few questions elicit symptoms of a clinical depression.

In the unlikely event that there is no marital or family therapy planned, we contact the significant other at least monthly via phone or in conjoint meetings. This provides an ongoing source of information about issues that arise and also serves to maintain whatever family plans were in place.

Education

The objective of this intervention is to reframe the presenting problems, validate and support the family, and motivate family members for further change. Didactic information groups where families learn about both chemical dependency and the psychiatric disorder, combined with sharing information and the impact these personal experiences have had on family members, are both crucial. Telling the secret, learning to attribute the damage to the twin illnesses, and finding out they are not alone are powerful experiences for many family members. We hold these sessions without the client present to permit an honest exchange of information.

We also encourage family members to contact appropriate sources for additional information. The National Alliance for the Mentally Ill has its national headquarters at NAMI, Colonial Place Three, 2107 Wilson Blvd., Suite 300, Arlington, VA 22201, 800-950-NAMI; and the National Mental Health Association is at 1021 Prince Street, Alexandria, VA 22314-2971, 800-969-NMHA. Alcoholics Anonymous General Services Office is at Box 459, Grand Central Station, New York, NY 10163, 212-870-3400; and Al-Anon Family Group Headquarters, Inc. is at 1601 Corporate Landing Parkway, Virginia Beach, VA 23454, 800-356-9996.

Support Groups

The objective here is to provide education, emotional support, and a start on working through the issues facing the family. Al-Anon, Alateen, and similar groups are excellent sources of support. Like members of Alcoholics Anonymous, participants in the Al-Anon family groups learn to work the Twelve Steps. They learn how destructive their attempts to control the uncontrollable are to themselves and others. Through the open sharing with other members they share experience, strength, and hope. They learn that they need and deserve help and begin their own personal recovery programs. Many of the lessons of Al-Anon apply to the psychiatric disorder as well. The concept of enabling, for example, is relevant to both groups. We like to supplement chemical dependency support groups with mental health support groups such as those run by the Alliance for the Mentally Ill. Parents and spouses of persons suffering from schizophrenia as well as other mental disorders share experiences and give support. Accepting that your loved one is mentally ill can be more difficult than accepting that he/she is an alcoholic. The stigma associated with mental illness can lead to guilt, fear, and feelings of loneliness for the family members of the mentally ill. A support group can be an excellent vehicle for learning acceptance and how to detach with love from the dually diagnosed family member. Ideally, the family can attend both kinds of meetings. If this is difficult, we prefer to emphasize the chemical dependency support groups, since we feel these will address key issues applicable to both.

Our experience is that family members who do embrace the Twelve Step philosophy ultimately do better. This occurs best when they attend meetings, but counselors can also tutor family members in recovery concepts from an Al-Anon perspective. Family members operating within this framework certainly are more willing to give up ineffective attempts to control the situation, to start with themselves and their part of the problem, and to let go of resentments and other emotional baggage. Family members also get practice talking about their feelings in meetings and, besides reactivating the ability to talk in this way, they burn off some of the strong affect that can prove a handful for counselors to manage in sessions. Having gone to Al-Anon meetings and worked the steps increases counselors' credibility and effectiveness here. This also will produce more realistic empathy for counselors who've not been in the situation of having to deal with a very troubled family member.

Behavior Management through a Home Behavior Contract

The objective during the early stages of recovery is to provide a safe, stable, and reasonably flexible environment for family members to lay the foundation for further growth. The focus is on giving the family a set of rules for responding to situations involving such things as threats of harm to self or others, failure to take medication, the resumption of chemical use, disobedience, and the failure of the dually diagnosed family member to follow through on the ongoing recovery program. We introduce the dually disordered person into family sessions when the client has some minimum level of stability, having preliminarily worked with the client and family separately. Families benefit from the establishment of reasonable rules to moderate extremes of chaos or rigidity and to begin to establish appropriate boundaries.

We make great use of contracts in this endeavor and supplement them with behavioral rehearsal in which family members practice implementing the contract. Not only does the contract provide a set of rules to govern family behavior, but the contract process gives families training in negotiating and problem-solving skills. Many families in early recovery tell us that the behavior contract was the only thing keeping the family sane during the early months of recovery. Appendix 4 presents a typical home behavior contract for adolescents and their families developed by our colleagues.

We would ask readers to note several features of the contract design. Some items refer to parental behavior and to treatment expectations for all parties. This communicates the message that change is expected of all family members. There are items that attempt to interrupt escalating exchanges and that shift the focus to positive behaviors. The longest time frame for Level 1 (the most severe) grounding is 72 hours. This gives the teens the incentive to comply because full privileges return quickly and it gets both the parents and the teens out of the no-win lockdown they typically have descended into. There is a lesser response cost for honestly reporting a relapse than for lying. Attending treatment when grounded to the property or the room even becomes a reward for the teen!

We sell the contract by framing it to all parties in ways that fit their world view. We might point out to the teens that they won't be grounded for weeks and talk to the parents about how they get to ground the teen several times a week and get back in control, for example. We then review the "goodies" of full privileges first to remind the teens what they have to gain for following the program. We then review the various expectations, complimenting all family members if items are not issues and removing them from the document, reviewing and negotiating pertinent items. Items can also be added as needed. We have all parties sign the contract and give them all copies. We then ask each family member where he/she might get off track in following the contract and problem solve any difficulties. Typically the contract takes one to two 1-hour sessions to negotiate.

Follow-up sessions focus on compliance with the contract by all parties and dealing with any problems that come up. Items can also be deleted, amended, or added as needed. For example, while consequences ideally occur as soon as possible after the infraction, parents may have difficulty monitoring a grounding during the week and might opt to implement this on the weekend instead, or we might challenge parents who fail to follow the contract.

Implementing the contract quickly identifies skill and process issues in the family. These can be addressed as needed, with the contract providing the overall frame. The therapist can prompt more skillful negotiating, pointing out to teens more "helpful" ways to request privileges. When impasses occur, we also might send either the teen or the parents out of the room for a brief mini-session to try to tone down unrealistic expectations or cool off too heated exchanges. We actively insist that something happen in the therapy session that is different from what happens at home.

We make use of written agreements with adults as well, although these are more general in tone and simply specify certain kinds of contingencies, such as agreeing to go to residential treatment if relapses continue.

In-Depth Work

As the family settles into a firm early recovery, its members are ready to begin in-depth work focused on further growth. More traditional family therapy approaches are suitable here. Information about child developmental issues can also be helpful, as are specific tasks designed to strengthen appropriate spousal, parent–child, and sibling relationships. A key set of tasks focuses on a fundamental need in these families, the need for fun. Families caught up in reactive, unhealthy systems never had the time or energy to play together. Families need to move from a problem-centered to a growth-centered existence. Practicing play behaviors helps them do this and also assists in establishing a positive emotional atmosphere. In this stage family members can also learn to work through and resolve old hurts, resentments, and wounds and move on with their lives.

SPECIAL ISSUES

The sequence of interventions discussed above is ideal and assumes a family is willing and able to work on its recovery. Needless to say, the counselor or case manager often faces a less-than-ideal situation. In this section we discuss some specific common dilemmas that providers encounter with dually diagnosed families and share some of our solutions.

Sometimes the family of a dually diagnosed client has severed all connections with him/her. This is especially true among adults with a mental illness. Sometimes a successful early recovery from both disorders sets the stage for a possible reunion, but this is not always the case. In these cases we focus on helping the client grieve the loss and move on with establishing a new life. At other times, the dually diagnosed client remains unmotivated for recovery despite our best efforts to break through denial and motivate him/her for change. We will not continue doing family work with the client if there is not significant abstinence or a minimum of psychiatric stability. We believe that this is a waste of time otherwise. We proceed instead by redefining our "client" as the family in these cases. At the very least, family members can enter recovery. Ironically, this sometimes prompts the client to start making positive changes.

Often the family feels that only the identified patient has a problem and that the service provider's job is to fix him or her. This "drop 'em off at the dry cleaners" attitude is frustrating for counselors, particularly since it removes access to important information and contingencies. These families respond to the suggestion that they need assistance with disbelief, anger, and resistance. In other cases an enabling spouse or parent rescues the client from treatment. Some providers and programs refuse to treat the client unless the family also participates, and this is certainly a viable option.

Counselors and case managers are more likely to obtain family cooperation if they do the following:

1. Make the final determination on who needs to attend, themselves, using input from the identified patient but reserving the right of final decision. Contact the family as early as possible and communicate, kindly but firmly, the expectation that they will participate.
2. Meet with the family as early as possible, ideally at the intake interview. Schedule family sessions then and there even if members have to call back to confirm.
3. Call the sessions "consultations" or some other term that avoids a blaming and judgmental focus and assure families that their involvement does not mean that clients are correct when they blame them for their problems.
4. Accept the family's goals and explain how the session can help to achieve them. For example, talk to the stepfather invested in getting things under control about how the home behavior contract will achieve this.
5. Have one therapist in charge of all contacts with both the identified patient and family whenever possible as the case manager. However, we also assign a separate family therapist that preserves the client's own individual therapy relationship and also allows for the possibility of therapists' playing "good cop, bad cop" now and then.
6. Position the therapists as experts with resources, and, whenever possible, do something useful for the family.
7. Communicate mainly through the family member who has the power to get the other members into the sessions. Sometimes identified patients are very powerful, and joining with them or making something they want contingent on family participation is useful. If one parent is ambivalent, contact the other parent. If parent and child are strongly allied, have them work on other family members. Putting the adolescent in charge of implementing the contract is an interesting intervention.
8. Provide family members an opportunity to talk about issues without the client.
9. Try to provide evening or weekend appointments and make provisions for young children.
10. Set up meetings with school officials, employers, and so forth to create social pressure for involvement. Arrange for frequent

reports to those with external power and remind the family that these other officials view family involvement favorably.

11. Have a receptionist call with a reminder of scheduled appointments, and, whenever family members miss a session, have the case manager contact the family by phone or letter.
12. Charge families for missed sessions.
13. Be sure to point out strengths frequently and compliment efforts to change.
14. Challenge family members to develop a more complex storyline for such family myths as "he's bad, we're fine."
15. With his or her permission, have a member of another family further along in recovery contact the family to share his/her "experience, strength, and hope."

Often another family member is also chemically dependent or psychiatrically disordered (or both). We are especially alert to depression and anxiety in the "codependents" as well as the current or recent history of substance use disorders. Getting other family members the treatment they need is important.

Sometimes family members are unwilling to do anything about their own problems. We handle this in a number of ways. Sometimes we have all family members take a Minnesota Multiphasic Personality Inventory (MMPI) and then meet individually with family members to go over the results and develop any needed action plan using "objective" data to increase the family member's insight. In the case of an adolescent we use the term "psychological emancipation" to describe the process of emotionally detaching from a dysfunctional parent. Sometimes we invite the family member to "clear up this issue one way or another" and attempt to get him/her to agree to an independent evaluation in or outside our clinic. The family member either feels less threatened or, if the situation blows up, the treatment of the identified client is more likely to be preserved.

Sometimes the family situation poses an immediate health and safety risk. Families where there is violence and abuse fit this category. When this risk exists and relevant laws exist, we report child or senior abuse or facilitate court commitment for mandated treatment and let the established system run its course. With adults we will recommend separation and the use of such resources as battered women's shelters and restraining orders. In cases where a family member shows a potential for possible harm to others, we will help the other family members to develop contingency plans that specify their responses to a dangerous situation. Examples include going to a relative's or neighbor's house when the other family member is drunk or threatening. Often family members are more willing to change during a crisis, and counselors and case managers can use this opportunity to help the family begin to work toward more permanent solutions.

Families of the dually diagnosed client need counseling and support. Involving the family in counseling increases the chances of a positive treatment outcome.

CHAPTER 11

Enhancing the Motivation of Clients (and Counselors, Too!)

Don't quit five minutes before the miracle.
—ANONYMOUS

Motivating clients for change is the key issue that providers of services to dually diagnosed clients face. The focus of this chapter is on enhancing the motivation of clients for dual recovery. We also briefly address counselor burnout.

MOTIVATION AND READINESS FOR TREATMENT

Stage Models of Change

Are there things that a clinician can do to enhance motivation? DiClemente and his colleagues have developed a stage model of change that appears to have both conceptual and empirical validity as well as clinical usefulness for conceptualizing changes in addictive behavior and probably for other behaviors as well (Prochaska et al., 1992). According to this model, the change process has five stages:

1. Precontemplation, where persons do not consider or do not want to change a particular behavior.
2. Contemplation, where persons acknowledge a problem and are considering a change.
3. Preparation, where persons plan to change soon and begin to take a few tentative steps toward change.
4. Action, where persons are actively changing or modifying behavior.
5. Maintenance, where persons sustain the changes, or relapse, when persons return to the earlier pattern of behavior and one of the first three stages.

Individuals can remain stable, progress, regress, or recycle through these stages.

Efficient change depends on persons doing the right things at the right time and on providers providing interventions matched to clients' stage of change. Two particular mismatches are common: trying to move into the action stage while relying on processes associated with only increased awareness; or trying to jump into the action stage without the awareness, decision making, and readiness provided by the contemplation and preparation stages.

Techniques appropriate to the precontemplation and contemplation stages include consciousness raising through such things as reading, classes, and visits to AA; dramatic relief through role playing, psychodrama, and expressing feelings about one's situation; and environmental reevaluation through such things as spouse meetings and empathy training. Techniques appropriate to the contemplation and preparation stages include self-reevaluation through such things as values clarification, a diagnostic workup with feedback to the client, and decision-making techniques, such as a listing of costs and benefits of a behavior; and self-liberation through such things as decision-making therapy, use of a helping relationship, and individual and group treatments. The techniques appropriate to the action and maintenance stages include reinforcement management, helping relationships, counterconditioning strategies such as relaxation training, and stimulus control tactics such as avoiding situations associated with chemical use. When relapse occurs, the challenge is to assist clients in avoiding being stuck or demoralized and to move back into the stage of contemplation or better.

Osher and Kofoed (1989) have outlined an influential stage model of motivation specifically for clients with dual disorders. They posit four stages:

1. Engagement, where providers work to convince clients that treatment has something of value for them.
2. Persuasion, a long-term process of attempting to convince clients of the need for abstinence.
3. Active treatment phase, where the emphasis is on developing skills and attitudes needed to maintain sobriety.
4. Relapse prevention.

Readers will note the similarities to the stages-of-change model just described. The Osher and Kofoed model served as the basis for the instrument called the "Substance Abuse Treatment Scale," (Drake et al., 1996), mentioned earlier (see Chapter 4). Readers will remember that clinicians can reliably rate their dually diagnosed clients as being in one of eight categories of recovery: preengagement, engagement, early persuasion, late persuasion, early active treatment, late active treatment, relapse prevention, and remission, or recovery. We are not aware of any research that systematically relates stages of change/readiness to treatment outcome at this time. Consistent with this model are treatment services that provide early intervention, pretreatment, or step zero groups that have the goal of helping clients in the early stages of treatment explore their concerns without requiring a commitment to action (Washton & Stone-Washton, 1991).

Conceptualizing change as a process and, further, giving specific referents and tactics for each stage makes this model a fruitful one for clinicians. We find that having experts acknowledge that some potential clients are not ready for change allows us to deal with our own codependence that tells us it's all up to us to have perfect clients. We also find support for many of the traditional interventions of substance use treatment, including education, attendance at support groups, and the telling of one's story. At the same time, we have been stymied whenever we used interventions that relied on cooperation with clients during the precontemplation stage of use. Clients will often state that they "might" have a problem and promise to go to a meeting and so forth. Yet, the next week comes and they haven't done anything. This move back into the precontemplation stage is most likely to occur if the crisis has passed that motivated an initial contact with services or if there has been some relief of one or both of the disorders. After several attempts to engage clients we will acknowledge the inevitable and arrange for discharge.

Life Event Factors Influencing Change

Why do those with substance use disorders decide to change? Alcoholics who consider themselves more seriously ill and who reported a higher incidence of recent negative events indicating a need for change in general and in regard specifically to their drinking are more likely to enter treatment or otherwise attempt to moderate or stop substance use than those who do not (Tucker, Vuchinich, & Gladsjo, 1994; Klingeman, 1991; Bardsley & Beckman, 1988; Krampen, 1989; Thom, 1987). One study found the following events, listed from most to least often cited by study participants, as prompting abstinence: illness or accident, extraordinary events (such as a suicide attempt or identity crisis), religious or conversion experience, alcohol-induced financial problems, intervention by immediate family, alcohol-related death or illness of a friend and intervention by friends (tied), education about alcoholism, and alcohol-related legal problems (Tuchfeld, 1981, cited in Kinney & West, 1996). Clients with substance abuse disorders specifically endorsed "weighing the pros and cons of drinking or drug use" and "a warning from spouse" as reasons for changing their use; and those who endorsed "hitting rock bottom," "weighing the pros and cons of drinking and drug use" and "major life-style change" were more likely to enter and stay in treatment in one study (Cunningham, Sobell, Sobell, & Gaskin, 1994). So-called coerced treatment, or treatment mandated by the legal system or employers, is a common prompt to entering therapy (e.g., Weisner, 1990).

The Therapeutic Relationship

Research has consistently found that the quality of the therapeutic relationship is an important factor in motivating substance-dependent and mental health clients (Bell, Montoya, & Atkinson, 1997; Connors, Carroll, DiClemente, Longabaugh, & Donovan, 1997; Najavits, Griffin, Luborsky, & Frank, 1995). Besides a user-friendly treatment system, high levels of therapist commitment to, and respect for, the client increase client retention in chemical dependency treatment services, as can providers' promoting the expectation that change is possible and treatment can help (e.g. Stark, 1992).

Miller and colleagues (Miller & Rollnick, 1991; Miller, Zweben, DiClemente, & Rychtarik, 1994) have focused on specific principles for use in the session with clients to enhance motivation to change their drinking. These principles include:

1. Give personalized feedback about the impact of clients' behavior on their lives.
2. Offer direct advice on how to change.
3. Provide a menu of options for how change might be accomplished.
4. Express empathy for the clients' situation.
5. Develop discrepancy by pointing out to clients the distance between their current status and their goals.
6. Avoid arguments.
7. Roll with resistance and defensiveness.
8. Support self-efficacy, the clients' sense of being able to cope with or manage a situation.

Providers espousing these principles attempt to join with and then maneuver clients rather than just confronting them head-on.

Contingency Management

Another approach to enhancing motivation is the use of contingency management techniques based on operant learning theory. Studies have demonstrated reductions in drug use and increases in treatment compliance by employing concrete rewards such as vouchers good for various rewards such as state lottery tickets, cash, access to disability payments, and even additional take-home doses of methadone (e.g., Iguchi et al., 1996). For probably obvious reasons, these interventions have focused to a large extent on stimulant and opioid drug abusers. The Community Reinforcement Approach (CRA) attempts to intervene to increase naturally occurring reinforcers for chemical-free behavior (Higgins et al., 1991; Hunt & Azrin, 1973). This has included arranging for assistance for obtaining jobs, arranging rewarding family interactions, and engaging in non-alcohol-related social activities. The original study even had a special social club with activities on Saturday nights, with admission dependent on abstinence. Another example is to arrange a pleasant activity with family members if the client remains sober. Operant procedures have also proven effective as mental health interventions for those suffering from schizophrenia and for children with conduct disorders, suggesting that they might also be appropriate, suitably modified, for dually diagnosed clients (Bigelow & Silverman, 1999; Shaner, Tucker, Roberts, & Eckman, 1999).

There are, however, clinical, financial, and political barriers to widespread implementation of contingency management strategies. Clients often switch to other drugs or illegal means of securing income, most programs not receiving special grant money couldn't afford these interventions, and many would object to either rewarding people for what they should do or attempting to coerce people in this way (Shaner et al., 1999). Lottery tickets may fuel a gambling addiction. Specific operant programs are costly and difficult to implement.

However, in a more general sense, quality treatment does attempt to help clients develop a lifestyle consistent with, and antithetical to, continued drug use and immobilization of psychiatric symptoms. Having fun in sobriety, managing negative emotions, and assisting clients in going back to school or obtaining work are all part of the habilitation and rehabilitation of clients. Research has demonstrated that treatment plans that are comprehensive and individualized in this way increase the effectiveness of dual diagnosis treatment (McLellan et al., 1997).

Intervening with Clients' Social Systems

Working with the social systems of clients is another way to enhance motivation. A formal intervention is one such strategy that involve family members and significant others to implement an intervention (Liepman, 1993). A trained professional works with the family for several sessions to educate members about substance use disorders, to allow them to ventilate their feelings, and to prepare a carefully scripted presentation of the impact of the loved one's substance use on each family member and the actions each is prepared to take if the loved one doesn't enter treatment. Participants also develop their own self-care plans. The goal is to both prompt treatment through a caring and coordinated confrontation of the alcoholic/user and to help other family members heal. The "moment of truth" of the intervention can break through the denial and result in entry into treatment. We have seen these techniques adapted for use with dually diagnosed individuals, including those with a coexisting bipolar disorder or anorexia.

At the same time, interventions can be a high-risk, high-gain strategy, especially with dually diagnosed clients. By raising the "bottom" that the addict or psychiatric client has to hit to "surrender," clients and their families can avoid the progression of the disease and enter recovery before things get even more out of hand. On the other hand, interventions can go quite badly, resulting in severe permanent damage to the relationships among clients and their significant others. Many families refuse to go through with the planned intervention. Clients can refuse to go into, or remain in, treatment. Family members can blame one another for this failure. Intervention can even provoke violence when families attempt an intervention with a volatile dually diagnosed client such as an individual with a paranoid schizophrenic disorder. Intervention with dually diagnosed clients requires an understanding of the interaction of the two disorders and careful preparation in order to avoid a disaster. Prior to planning any intervention, always consult with a trained expert. In the case of a dually diagnosed client, be sure to have a diagnosis of what the client's coexisting disorder is likely to be. Also use an interventionist familiar with both chemical dependency and mental health issues.

Network therapy (Galanter, 1993) and multisystemic therapy (Henggeler, Pickrel, Brondino, & Crouch, 1996) attempt to work with family members and significant others to become a team promoting abstinence and recovery. Providers focus on coaching the team members and also on strengths rather than on resolving areas of conflict, and team members, in turn, serve as monitors, implementers, and additional supports of targeted clients' treatment plans. Helping significant others resolve potential conflicts between being involved in the clients' treatment and Al-Anon's message of detachment with love is important for those involved in this 12-step program. We sometimes resolve this dilemma by making the distinction between reporting information to the therapist versus trying to be the therapist.

Suggestions Specifically for Dually Diagnosed Clients

Levy (1993) outlines an approach for clients with dual disorders whose substance use is not so extensive or life-threatening that immediate containment is the necessary provider response. He outlines a model that includes (1) helping clients find a treatment goal relevant to them; (2) over time, exploring the relationship between substance use and failure to attain the goal; (3) the therapist serving as the "observing ego" for the client to objectively help him/her make the connection between substance use and problems; and (4) drawing the link between symptoms and suffering and substance use as a well-meaning but failed solution.

Rosenheck (1995) discusses the responsible use of limit setting with dually diagnosed clients whose status requires such intervention. He outlines the following interventions: (1) verbal confrontation, where the clinician "vigorously" points out the destructive consequences of the behavior; (2) behavioral contracting, with specified conditions as requirements for continued treatment; (3) passive sanctions, when the provider withholds various kinds of assistance such as a referral to special housing; (4) invocation of external authorities, as in informing family members or probation officers; and (5) direct imposition of restrictions through such means as civil commitment or restricting access to funds by having a legally designated payee to manage the client's funds.

Daley and Zuckhoff (1999) outline principles for enhancing the treatment compliance of substance abusers and dually disordered clients. At the systems level they recommend such things as having a clear philosophy on compliance, providing staff training in strategies for motivating clients, providing reminders for appointments and callbacks for missed sessions, and employing consumer satisfaction surveys. They recommend many of the counseling strategies outlined above as well as such things as accepting ambivalence as normal, accepting and appreciating small changes, discussing current compliance problems immediately, and aggressively monitoring for signs of relapse.

A Two-Pronged Strategy and Some Specific Tactics

We have developed a number of our own strategies and tactics for enhancing clients' motivation. As noted earlier (in Chapter 3), we use flexible but direct challenges to clients' denial. In general we attempt to cultivate an attitude toward our clients of "*they're sick getting well, not bad getting good*," a phrase borrowed from Alcoholics Anonymous.

We also endeavor to implement a generic two-pronged strategy. The first prong involves efforts to *corral/contain* clients through the use of external systems such as family, schools, work, and probation/parole officers. The second prong consists of attempts to *align/join* with clients around their own goals, fears, desires, and needs. We keep in mind that, given that substance use disorders are rampant among clinical populations, our job is always to *rule out a substance use disorder, not rule this in,* for any client.

Specific tactics—some more, some less, important for managing denial and commitment to treatment—include the following:

• *Maintaining a user-friendly clinic setup.* This includes a comfortable, nicely appointed waiting room with fresh coffee, herbal tea, and hot-chocolate drinks, with current magazines available. The clinic is on a bus route, and we will subsidize bus passes from a special charity fund that has been created. Some of our younger "waif" clients actually "hang out" here, coming early and staying late, doing homework or just sitting. A separate room for children, stocked with toys and videos, is available off the main waiting area. After-hours, a "live" answering service takes messages and notifies the on-call clinician available for emergencies. Many clients tell us that they appreciate talking to a real person and not an answering machine for after-hours contacts. They also appreciate rapid access to a clinician in the event of an impending emergency. Clients receive reminder phone calls for all individual and family therapy appointments.

• *Scheduling intake appointments within 72 hours and much sooner if there is a full-blown crisis.* Our experience has been that waiting longer runs the risk of dissipating the positive momentum of any denial-reducing crisis.

• *Setting up the intake assessment in ways designed to increase its validity and ensure commitment to treatment.* Whenever possible, we talk with the referral source prior to the evaluation. This gives us the context for the evaluation and helps to inoculate us against the "denial" trance that clients can weave in the face-to-face interview through masterful use of thinking errors. We also screen insurance and other benefits so that we can problem solve possible financial barriers prior to seeing the client. We require a parent to accompany adolescents and strongly encourage adults to bring a significant other to provide collateral information and commitment to a treatment plan before ending the intake session.

Prior to our meeting, the receptionist staff obtains a routine set of releases for information that includes key collateral contacts such as parents, spouse, and primary-care physicians. Clients typically sign these without balking as part of the paperwork blizzard that intakes require and prior to any triggering of defensiveness in the session. We do verbally confirm with clients in the meeting the parties that we will contact for additional information and coordination.

Prior to interviewing clients, we meet briefly with all parties present to clarify the purpose, scope, reporting requirements, and limits to confidentiality of the assessment. We casually mention that a urinalysis is a routine part of our intake for all adolescent clients and for any adults where problematic substance use is a presenting problem and that a refusal is considered a "dirty" UA. We then inform all parties that we will meet first with the potential client and then separately with any significant other that has accompanied him/her and finally meet as a group at the end to determine the treatment plan. We do let clients know that we will not disclose all information that they tell us to collaterals but that we sometimes do have to inform particularly parents of any safety or health risks and that clients should let us know anything they don't want us to tell. We inform them that we will be happy to discuss this with them but that we reserve the right to make a final judgment about the degree of risk involved in any problematic behavior reported to us and the need to inform others.

• *Assessing external and internal sources of motivation at intake and throughout treatment and formulating goals that take these into account.* We inquire about the reasons for the client's coming for the assessment—its context and timing—with questions about what happened to get him/her here now. We inquire about incentives outside the client, such as an angry spouse, a pending legal charge of possession, or a suspension from school. We ask about the client's opinions about the events leading up to the intake to gauge internal incentives such as shame or an existential moment of clarity about life and death. We ask what clients would like to do more of and less of. We listen for implied goals—such as "to stay out of jail," "to save my marriage and job," "to be a better Christian"—and explicitly confirm these with clients. We later frame treatment recommendations in terms of these goals. We also listen with the proverbial therapeutic "third ear" for underlying worst fears and best hopes. For example, a client with narcissistic defenses values "looking good" above all else as a defense against underlying shame. These clients most fear looking foolish and being humiliated and most want the respect of others (typically the father in the case of males). Couching continued use in terms of humiliation and sobriety in terms of honor and respect can be helpful. A very common fear for many clients is that of being alone and unloved, and the wish is to belong and be loved. Formulating treatment to tap into this can garner some energy off these wellsprings of energy.

• *Developing a positive vision for the future and making frequent references to this throughout treatment.* This picture might be something like "being with my children again" or "having my own place." We invite clients to spend time—especially as part of Step 2-type interventions—in developing this picture in various ways. For example, we might invite the client to tell us how this vision looks, sounds, feels, even smells in great detail or have a client do a collage depicting this vision. We will attempt to help clients develop a realistic picture. We then constantly refer back to this picture in proposing interventions, and we pair dual recovery with achieving this goal.

• *Establishing the "helpful, hopeful expert" position.* We strive to maintain a collaborative but authoritative stance with clients. We want them to achieve their goals, and we know some excellent ways to help them do it. Waffling only increases anxiety and provides opportunities for denial to take over. Expressing firmly in words and tone "Keep coming back, it works" is important for activating hope and positive expectations.

• *Taking treatment as given and then offering choices whenever possible.* When presenting treatment recommendations to clients who are balky, we act as if the need for treatment is already accepted and focus the debate on whether the treatment, for example, should take place in a more restrictive residential environment (painted in less than rosy terms) or on an outpatient basis.

• *Sticking to "symptoms" and "behaviors" early on and avoiding premature labeling or diagnosing.* Such terms as "alcoholic" or "addict" are potentially explosive, and acceptance of the diagnosis, while helpful, is typically a long-term process.

• *Deliberately surfacing resistances.* At intake we specifically ask whether clients have any reservations or objections to what we are recommending and our rationale for this. At the end of sessions we ask clients if they have concerns about the session or the next treatment interventions on the schedule. We prefer to deal with these objections before clients walk out the door.

• *Attempting to get clients committed to a specific treatment plan and the next appointment prior to leaving.* Vague recommendations, or "think about it and get back to me," merely present opportunities for slipping away.

• *Mirroring the ambivalence through parts language.* We often use parts language to get beyond resistance. We might say something like "There's that part of you that thinks that people are just overreacting but there's that other part that wonders if there's really a problem." This kind of response doesn't corner clients and either expresses empathy or, in some cases, uses the power of suggestion to build up motivation for doing treatment.

• *Agreeing to disagree.* Sometimes mirroring the ambivalence can take place through saying something like "I know that you know we have different opinions about this. Let's talk some more."

• *Proposing the abstinence experiment.* If, in fact, chemicals are a take-it-or-leave-it proposition, then clients should have no trouble stopping use, or drinking only two drinks twice a week, say, for 30 days and then together examining what happens.

• *Being ready to do a mini-intervention.* While we prefer clients at intake to commit prior to talking to the significant other, sometimes our meeting time with the parents or spouses is spent doing a quick assessment on whether they are ready to institute a bottom line today with clients and, if possible, implement this. We do not proceed with this treatment, however, if we have any sense that the significant others will not defend the bottom line.

• *Having a designated case manager.* We feel it is crucial to have one person in charge of coordinating all information and treatment about each specific client. This is particularly important when several systems are involved because of the increased opportunities for playing parties against each other and paralysis. In our clinic the designated case manager is the person doing the individual therapy, but other arrangements are possible.

• *Generating a written treatment contract in the first session or so.* This is the opportunity to negotiate a plan that can engage clients. This can serve as a reminder to clients of their agreements if they get balky in later sessions. However, while we are willing to negotiate certain aspects of the plan, others are nonnegotiable. We might be OK, for example, with a client with moderate depression who does not want to take medication and go along with this as long as there is a willingness to reconsider the issue if depressive symptoms do not disappear over a 4- to 6-week period of time. This time frame and the backup plan are both added to the treatment plan. On the other hand, we will not accept a treatment plan that allows clients to "use whenever I want to" while they offer only to continue in treatment for their major depression. Contracts are more likely to be effective if they are specific, time-limited, achievable, and stated in terms of what the parties will do (rather than what they will *not* do), and, most importantly, specify consequences.

We have encountered frequent pitfalls in negotiating contracts with dually diagnosed clients. These include language that is vague, specifying consequences the provider cannot control, and inadequate access to data regarding client compliance. Other pitfalls include making exceptions to the contract's terms without explicitly renegotiating them and failing to get clients to agree explicitly and specifically to new terms of the contract.

• *Involving all relevant parts of the system as part of the "corral."* Families attend educational workshops and have joint therapy sessions where they complete, for adolescents, a written behavior agreement with specified consequences (as discussed in Chapter 10). At a minimum, frequent phone contacts with parents, spouses, schools, employers, probation officers and, if needed, "summit" meetings to review progress and any sustained failures to follow the treatment plan are helpful.

• *Labeling denial as a symptom.* When clients evidence denial, we simply state something like "Of course, you'd think it's OK to still drink even though you've had a problem with pot—that's how denial and addiction work." Then we go on to address the drinking issue as though the client has now accepted that this is a problem. Discussing with clients the thinking errors material contained in Chapter 4 is also helpful.

• *Using last-chance agreements.* We have "summit" meetings with clients who continually do not comply with the treatment plan, hoping thereby to work out a last-chance agreement. This agreement specifies the requirements necessary to remain in treatment or otherwise receive a referral for a more intensive level of care (as discussed in Chapter 5). Referrals are made not in a punitive spirit but in the spirit of a worsening of the client's illness and the need for more intensive treatment.

• *Making frequent reviews of progress and expressing praise and admiration for any positive changes.* In the spirit of Step 2, pulling back from the immediate stresses and reviewing for clients the progress they have made overall is helpful. Similarly, maintaining the "Progress not perfection" attitude embodied in the AA slogan helps with any black-and-white thinking about success and failure among both clients and providers.

• *Working to ensure a smooth referral from one care provider to the next.* This increases the likelihood the person will stay engaged in the continuum of care. In our experience clients are more likely to follow through with the treatment plan if they have a chance to meet their next provider and visit a site prior to entry into that system. Having an appointment for admission or a session already scheduled is also helpful. Phone calls or notes between providers indicating that clients are arriving and returning as planned help with compliance. This can alert providers to the start of trouble and can provide support for clients who know that their care "committee" is monitoring the situation, tracking their progress, and serving as a strong support system. Even within our own clinic we will try to take a moment to introduce clients to the therapist who will be doing their family therapy, for example.

• *Doing frequent case reviews of "stuck" clients in team and individual case supervision.* These weekly meetings achieve a number of goals. They can inspire new and fresh approaches to a case, spot clients falling through the cracks, head off team splitting, and, through repetition, train staff in motivational interventions and the clinic's policies and procedures for compliance.

DEVELOPING FAITH THAT RECOVERY IS POSSIBLE

Evans (1999) specifically set out to study the sources of motivation for change for one group of clients that she frequently works with. In her research with addicted adolescent female survivors of traumatic abuse, she found that positive transference between the therapist and clients can serve as a strong and key catalyst for change. By developing a positive helping alliance between the addict and the therapist, these addicts begin to adopt the therapist's belief that recovery can be achieved as an act of faith in the therapist. Clients initially change their behavior in order to please the therapist. With time, the clients begin to develop their own motivation for recovery and are able to transfer their faith in a "Higher Power" from the therapist onto a God of their understanding. Clients come "to believe that a power greater than [themselves can] restore [them] to sanity" (Alcoholics Anonymous, Step 2).

Evans found that successfully engaging clients in this change process and following through to success require several key ingredients:

1. Developing a rapport through initially joining with the client's world view and conveying empathy for his/her situation.
2. Creating an environment of trust by being reliable, keeping promises, and maintaining consistent boundaries.
3. Developing a "yes" mind-set by phrasing leading questions in a way designed to elicit an answer of yes from the client.
4. Identifying clients' sources of motivation for change and utilizing them as described above.
5. Aligning with the client's goals in contracting for change.
6. Acknowledging small steps achieved on the path of recovery.
7. Predicting success.
8. Adopting a "no failures, just lessons" philosophy.
9. Identifying high-risk relapse situations and problem solving them.
10. Rehearsing and "walking through" potential relapse scenarios to successfully get back on the recovery track.

While these 10 steps may seem obvious, cocreating a therapeutic environment for this change process to occur requires an accepting attitude on behalf of both therapist and clients. The magic for developing this atmosphere is quite simple: it is respect. Most addicts have much guilt and shame about their drinking and using behavior. They assume and project that the therapist is also going to see their behavior in a negative light. Providing a supportive, nonjudgmental atmosphere is the key to establishing a therapeutic alliance. By letting addicts see that you, the therapist, are a real person who also has made mistakes and that you are not sitting in judgment of them sets the tone for a positive therapeutic climate. Therapists who have a formal style may have more difficulty with this style of therapy, a style more typical of classic addictions counseling. This style takes on the tone of one addict helping another. This is not to say that clinicians who are not recovering cannot be effective, and it also does not mean that they should put on an act to try to seem hip, slick, and cool. The issue is genuineness.

MAINTAINING PROVIDER MOTIVATION

Providers also must sustain their motivation and not relapse into therapeutic pessimism. Keeping in mind that progress with dually diagnosed clients is slow but often steady helps with this. Providers will find it helpful to remember that many dually diagnosed clients, especially those with significant anxiety and depression, become quite motivated to maintain recovery once they get a taste of chemical-free living and recognize that they in fact feel worse when they use.

Despite our best efforts, however, some dually diagnosed clients refuse to enter treatment or end up leaving services prematurely. In these cases we sometimes proceed to redefine the client, preferring to work instead with the significant others who are often trying to cope with both the identified client and their own difficulties. We proceed by giving them information and referring them to support groups such as Al-Anon and the National Alliance for the Mentally Ill (NAMI). Engaging significant others in their own treatment is helpful to them and, ironically, sometimes results in the original client's reengaging in treatment. At other times we just have to accept that we have done the best we can do.

BURNOUT

Being alert to possible burnout is vital. Burnout is characterized by emotional exhaustion, depersonalization of clients, and a sense of inadequate personal accomplishment (Benbow, 1998; Gupchup, Lively, Holiday-Goodman, Siganga, & Black, 1994). Human services workers, including counselors of all persuasions, are very vulnerable to burnout (Felton, 1998). Increasing irritability, passive "whatever" counseling, and even sleep disturbance are some of the signals of burnout in providers. Clinical depressions are a possibility, as is the development of substance abuse (McKnight & Glass, 1995).

Simply acknowledging to oneself that burnout is occurring can go a long way toward keeping burnout from contaminating one's work. Hopefully the work environment is open to discussions of these feelings, and organizational norms do not idealize the "iron person" provider.

Many of us who have made our professional lifework the addiction field can become rigid and inflexible. We may find that we have slipped into trying to control clients' chemical use and other symptoms. We may fall into taking it personally if clients relapse. Clients may blame us for not being a good enough counselor to help them stay sober and stable. This can be a very toxic situation. If we start to doubt ourselves and our abilities, we have slipped into trying to control our clients' drug use. Addiction is a disease. It is a chronic disease. And relapse is common. Most psychiatric disorders are diseases, and relapse is also common. For dually diagnosed clients with two or more diseases relapses are completely predictable. We cannot allow ourselves to fall into thinking that we can control biological diseases. It is not helpful to personalize the challenges that all dually diagnosed clients have in staying sober and stable.

There is a saying in 12-step programs that goes like this: "We can carry the message, but we cannot carry the alcoholic." If we are taking too much responsibility for our clients' relapses and recoveries, then we have slipped into a subtle but potent enabling stance. If we are sweating harder than clients then we are taking the responsibility for the clients' behavior rather than having clients take responsibility for their own behavior. This is a set-up for conflict, counselor stress, and self-recrimination and, ultimately, counselor burnout. We need to "let go and let God." It is highly recommended that clinicians working with dually diagnosed addicts participate in Al-Anon. In that way we can utilize the peace and serenity that the 12-step program offers. Staying clear on boundaries and forgiving ourselves when we make mistakes not only prevents burnout but offers us an island of sanity in a sea of turbulent and challenging problems.

Strategically chosen days off, good self-care, and ongoing education are anodynes for burnout. Management can assist with allocating greater job control to workers, group meetings, flexibility in work assignments, and recognition of individual efforts. Developing career goals and a plan for achieving them is also useful in preventing burnout. And keeping realistic expectations of one's self, clients, and colleagues is crucial. Articles, workshops, and books citing interventions that are effective compared to other control conditions can create a misleading impression of the relative likelihood of actually "curing" clients. Certainly in working with dually diagnosed clients, some things work better than others, but providers are well advised to keep in mind that factors other than our interventions are much more powerful determinants of clients' prognoses and outcomes. Yet, we *can* make a difference—but only one day at a time.

Modified Stepwork

MODIFIED FOR THE CLIENT WITH PSYCHOSIS

Step 1

"We admitted we were powerless over alcohol; that our lives had become unmanageable."

Part 1

Please checkmark whichever of the following statements apply to you because of your drinking and using:

☐ People tell me I drink or use too much.
☐ Others get mad at me when I drink or use.
☐ I have tried to stop or cut back my drinking and using but started up again.
☐ Sometimes I drink and use more than I plan to.
☐ I have lost jobs or had to move after I have been drinking and using.
☐ I have ended up in the hospital after I have been drinking or using.
☐ I have been arrested after drinking and using.
☐ My drinking and using has caused me medical problems.
☐ I have spent all my money on alcohol and drugs.
☐ I have become more nervous and afraid at times when drinking or using.
☐ I have felt more distrustful and fearful of others after drinking or using drugs.
☐ My thinking is more confused when I drink or use.
☐ I have more trouble even doing simple things when I've been drinking or using.

Part 2

Give two examples of problems you now have because of your drinking and using.

Part 3

Give two examples of trouble you have gotten into in the past because of your drinking and using.

Part 4

Please checkmark whichever of the following statements apply to you because of your psychosis:

- ☐ My feelings are strange and all messed up.
- ☐ I have trouble thinking clearly and concentrating.
- ☐ Other people don't believe me when I tell them about the awful things that are going on.
- ☐ I am having strange experiences that others say can't be true.
- ☐ Lately I have trouble doing even simple things.
- ☐ I have to drink or use drugs to feel better.
- ☐ I feel sick a lot of the time, and I'm not sure why.
- ☐ Strangers talk about me and wish me harm.
- ☐ The only time I feel comfortable with others is when I drink or use.
- ☐ I have weird thoughts and feelings.
- ☐ The world has become a strange and frightening place.

Part 5

Give two examples of how your psychosis has made your life difficult.

Part 6

If you were taking medication for your psychosis and stopped, give two examples of problems that this caused you.

Part 7

What are some bad things that might happen if you were to continue to drink and use?

Part 8

How might things be more difficult if you don't take medication?

Part 9

Why might it be a good idea to take your medication?

Part 10

Why might it be a good idea to stop drinking and using drugs?

Step 2

"Came to believe that a power greater than ourselves could restore us to sanity."

Part 1

Give one example of how things are getting better since you stopped drinking or using.

Part 2

Give one example of how things are better since starting your medication.

Part 3

How has your drinking and using made your life worse?

Part 4

How has your psychosis made your life difficult?

Part 5

Give one example of someone who has been of help to you and explain how they were helpful.

Part 6

Give an example of one other person who might be helpful to you.

Part 7

How has following the advice of your counselors and doctor been helpful?

Part 8

How might things get even better if you continue to stay clean and sober?

Part 9

How might things continue to get better if you take your medication?

Part 10

How might things continue to get better if you stay in treatment?

Step 3

"Made a decision to turn our will and our lives over to the care of God, as we understood Him."

Part 1

Give one example of something that you now worry about and why worrying about this matter might not be helpful.

Part 2

Give an example of a person who you think is helpful to you or you could trust at least a little.

Part 3

How can it help you to "turn your worries over" or discuss this worry with the person you trust?

Part 4

How does medication help you with your worries?

Part 5

How does counseling help you with your concerns?

Part 6
What other people and situations in your life are helping you?

Part 7

What are some other things that might be helpful to you?

MODIFIED FOR THE CLIENT
WITH BIPOLAR DISORDER

Step 1

"We admitted we were powerless over alcohol; that our lives had become unmanageable."

Part 1

Give three examples (no more than 25 words each) of how you have gotten into trouble because of drinking and using.

Part 2

Give two examples (not to exceed 25 words each) of situations where you have drunk or used more than you planned or times where you lost control of your behavior when drinking or using.

Part 3

List three symptoms that have convinced you that you probably have bipolar illness.

Part 4

Give two examples of how your drug/alcohol use has made your bipolar illness worse.

Part 5

Briefly describe two ways that your bipolar illness has made the problems due to your drug and alcohol use worse.

Part 6

What unfortunate things could happen to you if you continue to drink and use? How will drinking and using interfere with the treatment of your bipolar illness?

Part 7

What unfortunate things might happen to you if you don't take your medication for your bipolar illness? How will failing to treat your bipolar illness make your drug and alcohol use unmanageable?

Part 8

Briefly give two examples of ways that you tried to continue drinking or using despite getting into trouble but that failed to stop the problems.

Part 9

Give two brief examples of ways that you tried unsuccessfully to manage your bipolar illness on your own.

Part 10

Why are staying clean and sober and taking your medication so important?

Step 2

"Came to believe that a power greater than ourselves could restore us to sanity."

Part 1

Checkmark whichever of the following mistakes in thinking have contributed to your continuing to drink or use:

☐ Excuse making
☐ Blaming
☐ Justifying
☐ Superoptimism
☐ Lying
☐ Threatening others
☐ Presenting a false image
☐ Building up myself
☐ Assuming things about others
☐ Thinking "I'm unique"
☐ Grandiose thinking
☐ Intellectualizing
☐ Hostile and angry outbursts
☐ Making fools of others
☐ Playing the victim
☐ Exaggerating
☐ Redefining
☐ Minimizing
☐ Ingratiating yourself with others

Part 2

List the errors in thinking that might have kept you from acknowledging your bipolar illness and the need for medication.

Part 3

Give two examples of how your drinking and/or drug use led you to feel crazy, more manic, or depressed.

Part 4

Give two examples of how your bipolar illness led you to use more drugs and alcohol despite the negative consequences.

Part 5

Give two examples of how your life has improved since you stopped drinking or using drugs.

Part 6

Give two examples of how your life has improved since taking medication and getting treatment for your bipolar illness.

Part 7

Describe a realistic positive picture of your life in the future as you grow in your dual recovery.

Step 3

"Made a decision to turn our will and lives over to the care of God, as we understood Him."

Part 1

Give two brief examples of how your bipolar illness and your addiction might improve if you found a way to "turn them over" to your Higher Power.

Part 2

Give one brief example (maximum of 50 words) of a situation where you tried to control someone else's behavior.

Part 3

How might your Higher Power have been more powerful and helpful than your own self-will in the situation you cited in Part 2?

Part 4

Give two examples of people who have been or could be helpful to you. Briefly describe how they have been or might be helpful (maximum of 25 words each).

Part 5

Give an example of a current problem you are having related to your addiction and mental illness. Describe how talking it over with a trusted person would strengthen your recovery and be helpful to you (maximum of 50 words).

Part 6

Who or what is your Higher Power?

Part 7

Describe how you might turn worries and concerns over to your Higher Power and how that might be helpful?

MODIFIED FOR THE CLIENT
WITH CLINICAL DEPRESSION
Step 1

"We admitted we were powerless over alcohol; that our lives had become unmanageable."

Part 1

Give three examples of how you have gotten into trouble because of drinking and using.

Part 2

Give two examples of situations where you have drunk or used more than you planned or times where you lost control of your behavior when drinking or using.

Part 3

List at least three symptoms that show that you suffer from major depression.

Part 4

Give two examples of how your drug/alcohol use has made your depression worse.

Part 5

Describe two ways that your major depression has made the problems due to your drug and alcohol use worse.

Part 6

What negative things could happen to you if you continue to drink and use? How will drinking and using interfere with the treatment of your major depression?

Part 7

How might things stay bad if you don't treat your major depression? How will failing to treat your major depression make your drug and alcohol use unmanageable?

Part 8

Briefly give two examples of ways that you tried to continue drinking or using despite getting into trouble but that failed to stop the problems that your drinking and using caused.

Part 9

Give two brief examples of ways that you tried unsuccessfully to manage your major depression on your own.

Part 10

How will staying clean and sober and treating your major depression with medication and/or counseling make things better?

Step 2

"Came to believe that a power greater than ourselves could restore us to sanity."

Part 1

Checkmark whichever of the following mistakes in thinking contributed to your continuing to drink or use:

☐ Excuse making
☐ Blaming
☐ Justifying
☐ Superoptimism
☐ Lying
☐ Threatening others
☐ Presenting a false image
☐ Building up myself
☐ Assuming things about others
☐ Thinking "I'm unique"
☐ Grandiose thinking
☐ Intellectualizing
☐ Hostile and angry outbursts
☐ Making fools of others
☐ Playing the victim
☐ Exaggerating
☐ Redefining
☐ Minimizing
☐ Ingratiating

Part 2

Describe the depressive thinking that discourages you from believing that your depression can get better with treatment and sobriety.

Part 3

Give two examples of how your drinking and/or drug use led you to feel crazy or more depressed.

Part 4

Give two examples of how your major depression led you to use more drugs and alcohol despite the negative consequences.

Part 5

Give two examples of how your life has improved since you stopped drinking or using drugs.

Part 6

Give two examples of how your life has improved since getting treatment for your major depression.

Part 7

Describe what has kept you going even during the bad times and how continuing to keep this in mind might help you now.

Step 3

"Made a decision to turn our will and our lives over to the care of God, as we understood Him."

Part 1

Give two brief examples of how your major depression, your addiction, and your life might continue to improve if you found a way to "turn them over" to your Higher Power.

Part 2

Give an example of a situation where you tried to control someone else's behavior.

Part 3

How might your Higher Power have been more powerful and helpful than your own self-will in the situation cited in Part 2?

Part 4

Give two examples of people who have been or could be helpful to you. Briefly describe how they have been or might be helpful.

Part 5

Give an example of a current problem you are having related to your addiction and major depression. Describe how talking it over with a trusted person would strengthen your recovery and be helpful to you.

Part 6

Who or what is your Higher Power?

Part 7

Describe how you might turn worries and concerns over to your Higher Power and how that might be helpful.

MODIFIED FOR THE CLIENT WITH AN ANXIETY DISORDER

Step 1

"We admitted we were powerless over alcohol; that our lives had become unmanageable."

Part 1

Give three examples of how you have gotten into trouble because of drinking and using.

Part 2

Give two examples of situations where you have drunk or used more than you planned or times where you lost control of your behavior when drinking or using.

Part 3

List at least three symptoms that show that you suffer from anxiety disorder.

Part 4

Write down the name of your anxiety disorder and then give at least two examples of how your drug/alcohol use has made your anxiety disorder worse.

Part 5

Describe two ways that your anxiety has made the problems due to your drug and alcohol use worse.

Part 6

What negative things could happen to you if you continue to drink and use? How will drinking and using interfere with the treatment of your anxiety disorder?

Part 7

How might things get worse if you don't treat your anxiety disorder? How will failing to treat your anxiety disorder make your drug and alcohol use unmanageable?

Part 8

Briefly give two examples of ways that you tried to continue drinking or using despite getting into trouble but that failed to stop the problems that your drinking and using caused.

Part 9

Give two brief examples of ways that you tried to unsuccessfully manage your anxiety disorder on your own.

Part 10

How will staying clean and sober and treating your anxiety disorder with medication and/or counseling make things better?

Step 2

"Came to believe that a power greater than ourselves could restore us to sanity."

Part 1

Check which of the following mistakes in thinking contributed to your continuing to drink or use:

☐ Excuse making
☐ Blaming
☐ Justifying
☐ Superoptimism
☐ Lying
☐ Threatening others
☐ Presenting a false image
☐ Building up myself
☐ Assuming things about others
☐ "I am unique"
☐ Grandiose thinking
☐ Intellectualizing
☐ Hostile and angry outbursts
☐ Making fools of others
☐ Playing the victim
☐ Exaggerating
☐ Redefining
☐ Minimizing
☐ Ingratiating

Part 2

Describe the fear-based thinking that discourages you from working a program of dual recovery one day at a time?

Part 3

Give two examples of how your drinking and/or drug use led you to feel crazy or more anxious.

Part 4

Give two examples of how your anxiety disorder led you to use more drugs and alcohol despite the negative consequences.

Part 5

Give two examples of how your life has improved since you stopped drinking or using drugs.

Part 6

Give two examples of how you life has improved since getting treatment for your anxiety disorder.

Part 7

Describe what has kept you going during even the worst times and how continuing to keep this in mind might help you to cope better now.

Step 3

"Made a decision to turn our will and our lives over to the care of God, as we understood Him."

Part 1

Give two brief examples of how your anxiety disorder, your addiction, and your life might continue to improve if you found a way to "turn them over" to your Higher Power.

Part 2

Give an example of a situation where you tried to control someone else's behavior.

Part 3

How might your Higher Power have been more powerful and helpful than your own self-will in the situation cited in Part 2?

Part 4

Give two examples of people who have been or could be helpful to you. Briefly describe how they have been or might be helpful.

Part 5

Give an example of a current problem you are having related to your addiction and anxiety disorder. Describe how talking it over with a trusted person would strengthen your recovery and be helpful to you.

Part 6

Who or what is your Higher Power?

Part 7

Describe how you might turn worries and concerns over to your Higher Power and how that might be helpful?

MODIFIED FOR THE ADDICTED SURVIVOR
Step 1

"We admitted we were powerless over alcohol; that our lives had become unmanageable."

Part 1

Describe briefly three situations where your drinking or using drugs led you to be unsafe.

Part 2

Give an example of how your drinking and using have made your trauma symptoms worse.

Part 3

Describe a situation when drinking or using drugs led you to hurt yourself.

Part 4

What is the most upsetting thing that you have done when you think about your drinking and drug use or something you did to get alcohol and drugs?

Part 5

Describe ways that you have tried to make drugs and alcohol work for you or to manage the consequences of their use but that have failed in accomplishing these purposes.

Part 6

Checkmark whichever of the following statements apply to you:

☐ I sometimes drink or use more than I planned.
☐ I sometimes lie about my drinking or using.
☐ I have hidden or stashed away drugs or alcohol so I could use them alone or at a later time.
☐ I have had memory loss when drinking or using.
☐ I have tried to hurt myself when drinking or using.
☐ I can drink/use more than I used to without feeling loaded.
☐ My personality changes when I drink or use.
☐ I have school or work problems related to my drinking or using.
☐ I have family and friend problems related to my drinking or using.
☐ I feel sick or ill when I stop drinking or using.
☐ I have legal problems related to my drinking or using.

☐ My drinking and using have led me to have medical problems.
☐ My life has more and more revolved around drinking and using.
☐ I have been unable to cut down or stop my drinking or using for a long time.
☐ I have done things that I am ashamed of when drunk or loaded.

Part 7

Checkmark whichever of the following symptoms of trauma apply to you:

☐ I have trouble relaxing and am always "on guard."
☐ I am very irritable and angry most of the time, often for no good reason.
☐ I have trouble concentrating.
☐ I have disturbing memories or dreams.
☐ I work very hard to avoid thinking about certain memories or I try very hard to avoid being in particular situations.
☐ I feel numb and uninterested in life.
☐ I cannot remember certain episodes or parts of my life.
☐ Life seems useless and without meaning.
☐ My sleep is often disturbed.
☐ Reminders of certain past experiences make me feel upset.
☐ I cannot trust people or my own feelings.
☐ I "check out" of my feelings, thoughts, and body.
☐ I feel unreasonably ashamed about myself and my actions.

Part 8

Describe ways you have tried to fix or manage your trauma symptoms that haven't worked.

Part 9

Describe ways your trauma symptoms have made your drinking and using worse.

Part 10

Describe how getting sober and safe is important for you and your loved ones.

Step 2

"Came to believe that a power greater than ourselves could restore us to sanity."

Part 1

Give three examples of how your drinking or using was insane (remember that one definition of insanity is to keep repeating the same mistake while expecting a different outcome).

Part 2

Describe how your trauma symptoms have made you feel crazy.

Part 3

Checkmark whichever of the following mistakes in thinking and actions you previously used in order to make your drinking/using and your trauma symptoms OK:

☐ Blaming
☐ Lying
☐ Manipulating
☐ Excuse making
☐ Minimizing
☐ Thinking I am unique or special
☐ Cutting oneself when angry

☐ Ignoring or pretending
☐ Intellectualizing
☐ Using angry behavior to control others
☐ Playing the victim
☐ Trying to be perfect
☐ Using even more alcohol or drugs
☐ Using food, sex, shopping, gambling, or work to feel better

Part 4

Now describe how these led you to be unsafe and actually made things worse.

Part 5

Give an example of something good that has happened because you stopped drinking or using. Give another example of something good that is likely to happen.

Part 6

Give an example of something good that has happened since you started dealing with your trauma symptoms. Also give an example of something good that is likely to happen.

Part 7

Who or what is your Higher Power and why do you think it can be helpful to you? Explain why coming to believe may take time and why that's OK.

Part 8

Are you angry at your Higher Power? If so, why? Do you feel unworthy of receiving help from your Higher Power? If so, why?

Part 9

Explain why it is important to find a Higher Power that you can trust, that you are not angry at, and that you feel worthy of receiving help from.

Part 10

Describe in detail a positive scene in the future that represents the you that will be sober and stable.

Step 3

"Made a decision to turn our will and our lives over to the care of God, as we understood Him."

Part 1

Explain why and how you decided to turn your will over to a Higher Power.

Part 2

Give two examples of things or situations you have turned over to your Higher Power in the past week, or give two examples of things you could have turned over.

Part 3

List two current resentments you have and then explain why it is important for you to turn them over to your Higher Power.

Part 4

What is one way you can turn over a resentment to your Higher Power?

Part 5

List two current worries or concerns that you have and then explain why it is important for you to turn them over to your Higher Power.

Part 6

What is one way that you can turn worries and concerns over to your Higher Power?

Part 7

Explain why you need to turn your will and life over to a power greater than yourself and how you are going about it.

Step 4

"Made a searching and fearless moral inventory of ourselves."

Part 1

List five specific things you like about yourself.

1.
2.
3.
4.
5.

Part 2

Give two examples of situations where you have been helpful to others since you have been sober and stable.

Part 3

Give three examples of behavior related to your drinking or using that you feel badly about.

Part 4

Give an example of behavior related to your trauma that you feel badly about.

Part 5

Describe how holding on to your own shame and guilt for your past behavior is not helpful to your dual recovery.

Part 6

Explain how working the first three steps can help you let go of unreasonable shame and guilt from the past.

Part 7

List two current resentments. Explain why holding on to these resentments hurts your dual recovery and how working the first three steps can help rid you of these resentments.

Part 8

List three new behaviors you have learned that are helpful to your dual recovery.
1.
2.
3.

Part 9

List two current fears you are experiencing and then discuss how working the first three steps can help dissolve these fears.

Part 10

Explain how being honest with yourself and others is important to your recovery.

MODIFIED FOR THE ANTISOCIAL CLIENT
Step 1

"We admitted we were powerless over alcohol; that our lives had become unmanageable."

Attach neatly printed answers to these questions on separate sheets of paper.

Part 1

Give five examples of ways you have tried to control your use of chemicals and have failed (minimum of 100 words each).

Part 2

Give five examples of people you have tried to control and have failed in doing so. Explain why your controlling behavior was unsuccessful (minimum of 100 words each).

Part 3

Give five examples of situations other than those associated directly with drinking or using that you have tried to control and have failed in doing so (minimum of 100 words each).

Part 4

Give two examples of people who currently have control over you, and explain how that is helpful to you (minimum of 100 words each).

Part 5

Give 10 examples (minimum of 25 words each) of how your drinking and using caused you problems.

Part 6

Give 10 examples (minimum of 25 words each) of how violating the rights of others or breaking the law caused you problems.

Part 7

Give five examples of negative consequences (minimum of 25 words each) that await you if you continue using drugs or alcohol.

Part 8

Give five examples of negative consequences (minimum of 25 words each) that await you if you continue breaking the law or violating the rights of others.

Part 9

Give five examples (minimum of 25 words each) of how your drinking and using helped you break the law or violate the rights of others.

Part 10

Give three examples (minimum of 25 words each) of how breaking the law or violating the rights of others helped you to continue your drinking and using.

Step 2

"Came to believe that a power greater than ourselves could restore us to sanity."

Attach neatly printed answers to these questions on separate sheets of paper.

Part 1

Repeating the same mistake over and over when you are constantly encountering negative consequences is one definition of insanity. From the list below, identify 15 major mistakes in your thinking. Explain with a minimum of 50 words each how this mistake in your thinking has caused your current problems.

- ☐ Excuse making
- ☐ Blaming
- ☐ Justifying
- ☐ Redefining
- ☐ Superoptimism
- ☐ Lying by commission, omission, or assent
- ☐ Making fools of others
- ☐ Playing the "big shot"
- ☐ Thinking "I'm unique"
- ☐ Ingratiating (yourself with others)
- ☐ Minimizing
- ☐ Intentionally being vague
- ☐ Using anger and threats
- ☐ Playing the victim
- ☐ Revelling in drama and excitement
- ☐ Not listening to others
- ☐ Maintaining a "look good" attitude
- ☐ Grandiose thinking
- ☐ Intellectualizing

Part 2

List three people you are currently angry at and explain how they could be helpful to you if approached correctly (minimum of 25 words each).

Part 3

List three people more powerful than you who can help you stay clean and sober. Explain why (minimum of 50 words for each person).

Part 4

Who or what is your Higher Power (minimum of 25 words)?

Part 5

Describe how this Higher Power can help you with your mistakes in thinking (minimum of 100 words).

Part 6

Describe how this Higher Power can help you respect the rights of others and obey the law (minimum of 100 words).

Part 7

Explain how this Higher Power can help you keep your freedom, your money, your relationships, and the respect of others (minimum of 100 words).

Step 3

"Made a decision to turn our will and our lives over to God, as we understood Him."

Attach neatly printed answers to these questions on separate sheets of paper.

Part 1

Why and how did you decide that you needed to turn your will over to a Higher Power (minimum of 100 words)?

Part 2

Why is it important for you to turn your will over to a Higher Power (minimum of 50 words)?

Part 3

Explain how you go about turning your will over to a Higher Power (minimum of 50 words).

Part 4

Give three examples of things you have had to turn over during the past week (minimum of 50 words each) and why this was good for you.

Part 5

Give three examples of things you have yet to turn over. Explain how and when you plan to do so and why this might be good for you (minimum of 75 words).

Part 6

What does it mean to turn your life over to your Higher Power (minimum of 100 words)?

Part 7

Without displaying any mistakes in thinking, explain why and how you have turned your life over to a power greater than yourself (minimum of 150 words).

Part 8

Without displaying any mistakes in thinking, explain in detail why turning your life and will over to your Higher Power is in your best long-term interest (minimum of 150 words).

Step 4

"Made a searching and fearless moral inventory of ourselves."

Attach neatly printed answers to these questions on separate sheets of paper.

Part 1

List any and all law violations you have committed, regardless of whether or not you were caught for these crimes (minimum of 100 words).

Part 2

List every person you have a resentment against and then explain how keeping this resentment is hurting you (minimum of 10 examples of 100 words each).

Part 3

Give 10 examples of sexual behavior you engaged in that was harmful to your partner, and explain the negative consequences to you of this behavior (minimum of 250 words).

Part 4

Give five examples of aggressive behavior (either verbally or physically) that you have been involved in, and explain how it was hurtful to the other person and how it was hurtful to you (minimum of 250 words).

Part 5

Give five examples of people you have ripped off (in terms of money, property, or emotions) and explain how it was hurtful to you and the other person (minimum of 250 words).

Part 6

List five major lies you have told, and then explain how that lying was hurtful to you (minimum of 250 words).

Part 7

List any and all lies you have told within the past 48 hours, and then explain how this lying hurts your recovery program (minimum of 200 words).

A School Behavior Checklist

Name of student: _____

Teacher or Counselor: _____

Class: _____ Period: _____ Date of report: _____

Please checkmark the following statements that apply to your observations of this student.

☐ Is tardy to class
☐ Is absent from three or more classes per term
☐ Seems disinterested in school work
☐ Appears apathetic and unmotivated to complete assignments
☐ Looks tired or sleepy in class
☐ Hands in assignments late
☐ Is not completing assignments
☐ Looks bored in class
☐ Seems overly restless in class
☐ Appears spaced-out in class
☐ Is disruptive in class
☐ Is hanging out with negative peers
☐ Appears to be changing peer groups to more negative ones
☐ Has lost interest in school activities
☐ Draws drug symbols and signs on papers or clothes
☐ Appears angry and guarded
☐ Looks sad or depressed
☐ Is easily irritated
☐ Is more moody than usual

☐ Has become more defiant toward authority
☐ Defends the use of drugs
☐ Defends the use of, or seems more intrigued by, violence
☐ Has been suspended one or more times in the past year
☐ Is underachieving, especially compared to past school performance
☐ Is getting into fights with other students

How long have you seen this behavior? _____

Is this a recent or sudden change in this student's behavior? _____

Comments:

Other concerns or important information that we should know:

A Checklist for Parents

HOW TO KNOW IF YOUR CHILD IS USING DRUGS

Your child may be involved in using drugs or alcohol if three or more of the following statements apply:

- Isolates him/herself more than before
- Is more argumentative with family members
- Is much more oppositional and challenging of family rules
- Is more secretive about where he/she is going and what he/she is doing
- Hangs around with an older group of friends
- Sees different friends than before
- Skips class three or more times per term
- Is experiencing a drop in grades
- Is much more distant and detached from family members
- Is feeling restless and "bored" all the time
- Is no longer interested in previously enjoyed activities
- Has had contact with the police or juvenile authorities
- Is in possession of money not easily explained
- Takes money and objects from other family members
- Money is mysteriously missing from around the house
- Displays a more severe "I don"t care" attitude than before
- Has experienced a substantial change in sleeping habits
- Has experienced a substantial change in eating habits
- Seems less interested in achievement and the future
- Defends the use of drugs
- Smokes cigarrettes regularly
- Wears clothing that contains slogans or symbols promoting drug use

A Typical Home Behavior Contract

This contract is meant to be used as a sample only. Items not relevant should be deleted. Do not use this contract with youth 17 or older unless the youth is presenting severe behaviors that require such restrictions. Instead use a behavior agreement limited to major items and more general consequences.

HOME BEHAVIOR CONTRACT FOR:

_____

Level System

LEVEL I: Room restriction for 24 hours unless otherwise specified below. _____ must stay in his/her room unless at school, doing required chores, or attending AA/NA meetings or therapy. There are no privileges at this level (including telephone, TV, radio, computer, etc.) Twenty-four hours of compliant behavior and a cooperative attitude warrant a level increase to Level II unless otherwise specified in demotion levels. Must go to Level II next and not skip ahead to Level III.

LEVEL II: On property. Does generally have other privileges (specify):
Must complete a work task to parent(s)' satisfaction and have 24 hours of compliant behavior and cooperative attitude in order to move to Level III. Parents will determine the work task at the time.

LEVEL III: Full-privilege status—VCR movies, theater movies, visit at a friend's home (time limit determined by parents), special family events, spending the night at a friend's home, driving privileges (and other privileges—specify):

_____

Demotion Levels

Listed below are the standard demotion levels. We suggest that Level I never exceed 72 hours total even for multiple infractions. Parents should drop levels as soon as possible. Any of the following behaviors will result in a drop in status as follows:

- Level I for 72 hours   Dirty urinalysis; chemical use, lying about use

                                         Runaway (AWOL; not in bed at lights out)

                                         Breaking the law

                                         Physical abuse

- Level I for 24 hours   Stealing

                                         Physical threats

- Level drop for 24 hours   Failure to follow other contract provisions

                                         Verbal abuse

                                         Lying in general

                                         Relapse in drug/alcohol use, honestly reported (and increased 12-step meetings, per counselor)

                                         School behavior problems (all problems in one day counted as one infraction)

                                         Persistent negative attitude

Behavioral Expectations

Home Schedule	Weekday	Weekend
Level I	Room restriction _____	Room restriction _____
Level II	Phone curfew _____ Lights out _____	Phone curfew _____ Lights out _____
Level III	Friend curfew _____ Phone curfew _____ Lights out _____ Home curfew _____	Friend curfew _____ Phone curfew _____ Lights out _____ Home curfew _____

1. _____ will not use mood-altering substances, except those prescribed by a physician.

2. No verbal abuse is permitted. Family members will make a reasonable effort to state assertively how they feel to other family members. Name-calling, screaming, yelling, etc., are not appropriate.

3. Homework must be done without arguing, completely, and on time. Parent(s) will set up a monitoring system with the school.

4. Assigned chores will be completed (per attached written schedule).

5. _____ will not engage in physical abuse, threats, or intimidation tactics.

6. _____ will not steal nor use other family members' possessions without permission.

7. _____ will not be late for chores, coming home from school, to meals, or to any expected activity. In case of any exception, he/she must call home prior to the time due for permission to come home at a later time.

8. _____ will not engage in inappropriate teasing and fighting with brothers and sisters.

9. _____ will accept "no" for an answer without arguing. Parents will provide a brief explanation of the reason for the "no." _____ may give a brief rebuttal (less than 3 minutes), but a second "no" is final.

10. All activities and friends must have the approval of parents. _____ may bring this item up for further discussion at a family therapy session.

11. Parents agree to focus on positive behaviors that _____ does and to decrease nagging, harping, "reminding." Parental compliance will be discussed in family therapy sessions.

12. Parents and _____ agree to plan and participate in a family activity together at least twice a month.

13. Parents may ask _____ to do up to 2 hours a week of additional tasks to contribute to the running of the home.

14. Parents will call the family counselor if there is a disagreement in the interpretation of the contract. _____ will follow the parental interpretation until that time.

15. Parents will call the family therapist or on-call counselor for a consultation if _____'s behavior is unsafe or escalating.

Treatment Contract

Teen's Part

1. _____ agrees to provide a good urine sample for urinalysis upon request by either the parent(s) or the outpatient therapists.

2. _____ will attend, be on time, and participate in:
   a. _____ number of individual sessions per week with _____
   b. _____ group therapy sessions per week, including (list groups):

   _____

3. _____ will attend 1–4 AA/NA meetings (specify number) _____ per week, per recommendation of the individual counselor.

4. _____ and other family members will attend family counseling with _____ as scheduled. Any family member can request a family therapy session.

Parents' Part

1. Parents will attend at least one Parent Education Group (may attend more).

2. Parents will attend at least three Al-Anon meetings prior to the end of treatment.

WITH OUR SIGNATURES BELOW, WE AGREE TO FOLLOW ALL THE RULES, EXPECTATIONS, AND CONSEQUENCES OF THIS HOME BEHAVIOR CONTRACT.

Teen   Date

_____   _____

Family Members   Date

_____   _____

_____   _____

Family Therapist   Date

_____   _____

References

Albanese, M. J., Barter, R. L., Bruno, R. F., Morgenbesser, M. W., & Schatzberg, A. F. (1994). Comparison of measures used to determine substance abuse in an inpatient psychiatric population. *American Journal of Psychiatry, 151,* 1077–1078.

Alcoholics Anonymous. (1957). *Alcoholics Anonymous comes of age.* New York: Alcoholics Anonymous World Services.

Alcoholics Anonymous. (1976). *Alcoholics Anonymous: The story of how many thousands of men and women have recovered from alcoholism* (3rd ed.). New York: Alcoholics Anonymous.

Alexander, P. C. (1992). Application of attachment theory to the study of sexual abuse. *Journal of Consulting and Clinical Psychology, 60,* 174–184.

Allen, D. M. (1997). Techniques for reducing therapy-interfering behavior in patients with borderline personality disorder: Similarities in four diverse treatment paradigms. *Journal of Psychotherapy Practice and Research, 6,* 25–35.

Allen, D. N., Goldstein, G., & Seaton, B. E. (1997). Cognitive rehabilitation of chronic alcohol abusers. *Neuropsychology Review, 7,* 21–39.

Alterman, A. I., McDermott, P. A., Cacciola, J. S., Rutherford, M. J., Boardman, C. R., McKay, J. R., & Cook, T. G. (1998). A typology of antisociality in methadone patients. *Journal of Abnormal Psychology, 107,* 412–422.

American Psychiatric Association. (1987). *Diagnostic and statistical manual of mental disorders* (3rd ed., rev.). Washington, DC: Author.

American Psychiatric Association. (1994). *Diagnostic and statistical manual of mental disorders* (4th ed.). Washington, DC: Author.

American Society of Addiction Medicine. (1996). *Patient placement criteria for the treatment of substance-related disorders* (2nd ed.). Chevy Chase, MD: Author.

Annis, H. M. & Davis, C. C. (1989). Relapse prevention. In R. K. Hester & W. R. Miller (Eds.), *Handbook of alcoholism treatment approaches* (pp. 170–182). New York: Pergamon Press.

Anthony, J. C., Warner, L. A., & Kessler, R. C. (1994). Comparative epidemiology of dependence of tobacco, alcohol, controlled substances, and inhalants: Basic findings from the National Comorbidity Survey. *Experimental and Clinical Psychopharmacology, 2,* 244–268.

Arndt, S., Tyrrell, G., Flaum, M., & Andreasen, N. C. (1992). Comorbidity of substance abuse and schizophrenia: The role of pre-morbid adjustment. *Psychological Medicine, 22,* 379–388.

Arntz, A. (1994). Treatment of borderline personality disorder: A challenge for cognitive-behavioral therapy. *Behaviour Research and Therapy, 32,* 419–430.

Ashton, H. (1995). Protracted withdrawal from benzodiazepines: The post withdrawal syndrome. *Psychiatric Annals, 25,* 174–179.

Ayuso-Gutierrez, J. L., & del Rio Vega, J. M. (1997). Factors influencing relapse in the long-term course of schizophrenia. *Schizophrenia Research, 28,* 199–206.

Azrin, N. H., and Teichner, G. (1998). Evaluation of an instructional program for improving medication compliance for chronically mentally ill outpatients. *Behaviour Research and Therapy, 36,* 849–861.

Babor, T. F., Brown, J., & DelBoca, F. K. (1990). Validity of self-reports in applied research on addictive behaviors: Fact or fiction? *Behavioral Assessment, 12,* 5–31.

Bardsley, P. E., & Beckman, L. J. (1988). The health belief model and entry into alcoholism treatment. *International Journal of Addictions, 23,* 19–28.

Barkley, R. A., Edwards, G. H., & Robin, A. L. (1999). *Defiant teens: A clinician's manual for assessment and family intervention.* New York: Guilford Press.

Barlow, D. H., & Lehman, C. L. (1996). Advances in the psychosocial treatment of anxiety disorders: Implications for National Health Care. *Archives of General Psychiatry, 53,* 727–735.

Bartels, S. J., Teague, G. B., Drake, R. E., Clark, R. E., Bush, P. W., & Noordsy, D. L. (1993). Substance abuse in schizophrenia: Service utilization and costs. *Journal of Nervous and Mental Disease, 181,* 227–232.

Basoglu, M., Marks, I. M., Kilic, C., Rewin, C. R., & Swinson, R. P. (1994). Alprazolam and exposure for panic disorder with agoraphobia: Attribution of improvement to medication predicts subsequent relapse. *British Journal of Psychiatry, 164,* 652–659.

Baucom, D. H., Shoham, V., Mueser, K. T., Daiuto, A. D., & Stickle, T. R. (1998). Empirically supported couple and family interventions for marital distress and adult mental health problems. *Journal of Consulting and Clinical Psychology, 66,* 53–88.

Bayatpour, M., Wells, R. D., & Holford, S. (1992). Physical and sexual abuse as predictors of substance use and suicide among pregnant teenagers. *Journal of Adolescent Health, 13,* 128–132.

Beach, S. R. H., & O'Leary, K. D. (1992). Treating depression in the context of marital discord: Outcome and predictors of response for marital therapy vs. cognitive therapy. *Behavior Therapy, 23,* 507–528.

Beattie, M. (1987). *Codependent no more.* New York: Harper/Hazelden.

Beatty, W. W., Katzung, V. M., Moreland, V. J., & Nixon, S. J. (1995). Neuropsychological performance of recently abstinent alcoholics and cocaine abusers. *Drug and Alcohol Dependence, 37,* 247–253.

Begleiter, H., & Kissin, B. (Eds.). (1995). *The genetics of alcoholism.* New York: Oxford University Press.

Bell, D. C., Montoya, I. D., & Atkinson, J. S. (1997). Therapeutic connection and client progress in drug abuse treatment. *Journal of Clinical Psychology, 53*, 215–224.

Benbow, S. M. (1998). Burnout: Current knowledge and relevance to old age psychiatry. *International Journal of Geriatric Psychiatry, 13*, 520–526.

Bierderman, J., Wilens, T., Mick, E., Milberger, S., Spencer,T. J., & Faraone, S. V. (1995). Psychoactive substance use disorders in adults with attention deficit hyperactivity disorder (ADHD): Effects of ADHD and psychiatric comorbidity. *American Journal of Psychiatry, 152*, 1652–1658.

Bigelow, G. E., & Silverman, K. (1999). Theoretical and empirical foundations of contingency management treatments for drug abuse. In S. T. Higgins & K. Sliverman (Eds.), *Motivating behavior change among illicit-drug abusers: Research on contingence management interventions* (pp. 15–31). Washington, DC: American Psychological Association.

Black, C. (1991). *It will never happen to me.* New York: Ballantine Books.

Blais, M. A., Hilsenroth, M. J., & Castlebury, F. D. (1997). Content validity of the DSM-IV borderline and narcissistic personality disorder criteria sets. *Comprehensive Psychiatry, 38*, 31–37.

Boney-McCoy, S., & Finkelhor, D. (1996). Is youth victimization related to trauma symptoms and depression after controlling for prior symptoms and family relationships?: A longitudinal, prospective study. *Journal of Consulting and Clinical Psychology, 64*, 1406–1416.

Bongar, B. (1991). *The suicidal patient: Clinical and legal standards of care.* Washington, DC: American Psychological Association.

Braun, B. G. (1988). The Bask model of dissociation. *Dissociation, 1*, 4–23.

Bremner, J. D., Randall, P., Scott, T. M., Capelli, S., Delaney, R., McCarthy, G., & Charney, D. S. (1995). Deficits in short-term memory of adult survivors of childhood abuse. *Psychiatry Research, 59*, 97–107.

Brennan, P. L., & Moos, R. H. (1990). Life stresssors, social resources and late-life problem drinking. *Psychology and Aging, 5*, 491–501.

Breslau, N., Davis, G. C., & Andreski, P. (1995). Risk factors for PTSD-related traumatic events: A prospective analysis. *American Journal of Psychiatry, 152*, 529–535.

Breslau, N., Davis, G. C., Peterson, E. L., & Schultz, L. (1997). Psychiatric sequelae of posttraumatic stress disorder in women. *Archives of General Psychiatry, 54*, 81–87.

Breslin, N. A. (1992). Treatment of schizophrenia: Current practice and future promise. *Hospital and Community Psychiatry, 43*, 877–885.

Briere, J., & Runetz, M. (1988). Symptomatology associated with sexual victimization in a nonclinical adult sample. *Child Abuse and Neglect, 112*, 51–59.

Brodsky, B. S., Clioter, M., & Dulit, R. A. (1995). Relationship of dissociation to self-mutilation and childhood abuse in borderline personality disorder. *American Journal of Psychiatry, 152*, 1788–1792.

Brown, G. R., & Anderson, B. (1991). Psychiatric morbidity in adult inpatients with childhood histories of sexual and physical abuse. *American Journal of Psychiatry, 148*, 55–61.

Brown, R. A., Evans, D. M., Miller, I. W., Burgess, E. S., & Mueller, T. I. (1997). Cognitive-behavioral treatment for depression in alcoholism. *Journal of Consulting and Clinical Psychology, 65,* 715–726.

Brown, R. A., Monti, P. M., Myers, M. G., Martin, R. A., Rivinus, T., Dubreuil, M. E., & Rohsenow, D. J. (1998). Depression among cocaine abusers in treatment: Relation to cocaine and alcohol use and treatment outcome. *American Journal of Psychiatry, 155,* 220–225.

Brown, S. A., Gleghorn, A., Schuckit, M. A., Myers, M. G., & Mott, M. A. (1996). Conduct disorder among adolescent alcohol and drug abusers. *Journal of Studies on Alcohol, 57,* 314–324.

Brown, S. A., Inaba, R. K., Gillin, C., Schuckit, M. A., Steward, M. A., & Irwin, M. R. (1995). Alcoholism and affective disorder: Clinical course of depressive symptoms. *American Journal of Psychiatry, 152,* 45–52.

Brunnette, M. F., Mueser, K. T., Xie, H., & Drake, R. E. (1997). Relationships between symptoms of schizophrenia and substance abuse. *Journal of Nervous and Mental Disease, 185,* 13–20.

Buchanan, J. (1995). Social support and schizophrenia: A review of the literature. *Archives of Psychiatric Nursing, 9,* 68–76.

Buchanan, R. W., Brerier, A., Kirkpatrick, B., Ball, P., & Carpenter, W. T. (1998). Positive and negative symptom response to clozapine in schizophrenic patients with and without the deficit syndrome. *American Journal of Psychiatry, 155,* 751–760.

Bukstein, O. G. (1995). *Adolescent substance abuse: Assessment, prevention and treatment.* New York: Wiley.

Burke, J. D., Jr., Burke, K. C., & Rae, D. S. (1994). Increased rates of drug abuse and dependence after onset of mood or anxiety disorders in adolescence. *Hospital and Community Psychiatry, 45,* 451–455.

Busto, U. E., Romanch, M. K., & Sellers, E. M. (1996). Multiple drug use and psychiatric comorbidity in patients admitted to the hospital with severe benzodiazepine dependence. *Journal of Clinical Psychopharmacology, 16,* 51–57.

Butzlaff, R. L., & Hooley, J. M. (1998). Expressed emotion and psychiatric relapse. *Archives of General Psychiatry, 55,* 547–552.

Byrne, A., Kirby, B., Zibin, T., & Ensminger, S. (1991). Psychiatric and neurological effects of chronic solvent abuse. *Canadian Journal of Psychiatry, 36,* 735–738.

Cacciola, J. S., Rutherford, M. J., Alterman, A. I., & Snider, E. C. (1994). An examination of the diagnostic criteria for antisocial personality disorder in substance abusers. *Journal of Nervous and Mental Disease, 182,* 517–523.

Cadoret, R. J., Yates, W. R., Troughton, E., Woodworth, G., & Stewart, M. A. (1995). Genetic-environmental interaction in the genesis of aggressivity and conduct disorders. *Archives of General Psychiatry, 52,* 916–924.

Cardone, A. A. (1995). Risperidone: Review and assessment of its role in the treatment of schizophrenia. *Annals of Pharmacotherapy, 29,* 160–168.

Carpenter, K. M., & Hittner, J. B. (1997). Cognitive impairment among the dually-diagnosed: Substance abuse history and depressive symptom correlates. *Addiction, 92,* 747–759.

Carpenter, W. T., Buchanan, R. W., Kirkpatrick, B., & Breier, A. F. (1999). Diazepam treatment of early signs of exacerbation in schizophrenia. *American Journal of Psychiatry, 156*(2), 299–303.

Carroll, K. M. (1996). Relapse prevention as a psychosocial treatment: A review of controlled clinical trials. *Clinical and Experimental Psychopharmacology, 4,* 46–54.

Carroll, K. M., Nich, C., & Rounsaville, B. J. (1995). Differential symptom reduction in depressed cocaine abusers treated with psychotherapy and pharmacotherapy. *Journal of Nervous and Mental Disease, 183,* 251–259.

Carroll, K. M., & Rounsaville, B, J. (1993). History and significance of childhood attention deficit disorder in treat-seeking cocaine abusers. *Comprehensive Psychiatry, 34,* 75–82.

Castenada, R., Sussman, N., Westreich, L., Levy, R., & O'Malley, M. (1996). A review of the effects of moderate alcohol intake on the treatment of anxiety and mood disorders. *Journal of Clinical Psychiatry, 57,* 207–212.

Catalano, R. F., Hawkins, J. D., Wells, E. A., Miller, J., & Brewer, D. (1990–1991). Evaluation of the effectiveness of adolescent drug abuse treatment, assessment of the risks for relapse and promising approaches for relapse prevention. *International Journal of Addiction, 25,* 1085–1140.

Caton, C. L. M, Wyatt, R. J., Felix, A., Grunber, J., & Dominguez, B. (1993). Follow-up of chronically homeless mentally ill men. *American Journal of Psychiatry, 150,* 1639–1642.

Chassin, L., Curran, P. J., Hussong, A. M., & Colder, C. R. (1996). The relation of parent alcoholism to adolescent substance use: A longitudinal follow-up study. *Journal of Abnormal Psychology, 105,* 70–80.

Childress, A. R., Hole, A. V., Ehrman, R. N., & Robbins, S. J. (1993). Cue reactivity and cue reactivity interventions in drug dependence. In L. S. Onken, J. D. Blaine, & J. J. Boren (Eds.), *Behavioral treatments for drug abuse and dependence* (NIDA Research Monograph Services No. 137, NIH Publication No. 93–3684). Rockville, MD: National Institute on Drug Abuse.

Christie, C., & Mitchell, S. (2000). *The addicted brain.* Jacksonville, FL: Professional Development Resources.

Christie, K. A., Burke, J. D., Regier, D. A., Rae, D. S., Boyd, J. H., & Loure, B. Z. (1988). Epidemiological evidence of early onset of mental disorders and higher risk of drug abuse in young adults. *American Journal of Psychiatry, 145,* 971–975.

Ciraulo, D. A., Barnhill, J. G., Ciraulo, A. M., Sarid-Segal, O., Knapp, C., Greenblatt, D. J., & Shader, R. I. (1997). Alterations in pharmacodynamics of anxioloytics in abstinent alcoholic men: Subjective responses, abuse liability and electroencephalographic effects of alprazolam, diazepam and buspirone. *Journal of Clinical Pharmacology, 37,* 64–73.

Clark, D. C., Gillin, J. C., Golshan, S., Demodena, A., Smith, T. L., Danowski, S., Irwin, M., & Schuckit, M. (1998). Increased REM sleep density at admission predicts relapse by three months in primary alcoholics with a lifetime diagnosis of secondary depression. *Biological Psychiatry, 43,* 601–607.

Clark, R. E. (1994). Family costs associated with severe mental illness and substance abuse. *Hospital and Community Psychiatry, 45,* 808–813.

Clarkin, J. F., Pilkonis, P. A., & Magruder, K. M. (1996). Psychotherapy of depression: Implications for reform of the health care system. *Archives of General Psychiatry, 53,* 717–723.

Connors, G. J., Carroll, K. M., DiClemente, C. C., Longabaugh, R., & Donovan, D. M. (1997). The therapeutic alliance and its relationship to alcoholism treatment and participation. *Journal of Consulting and Clinical Psychology, 65,* 588–598.

Conte, J. R., & Shuerman, J. (1987). The effects of sexual abuse on children: A multidimensional view. *Journal of Interpersonal Violence, 2,* 380–390.

Cornelius, J. R., Salloum, I. M., Ehler, J. G., Jarrett, P. J., Cornelius, M. D., Perel, J. M., Thase, M. E., & Black, A. (1997). Fluoxetine in depressed alcoholics. A double-blind, placebo-controlled trial. *Archives of General Psychiatry, 54,* 700–705.

Cornelius, J. R., Salloum, I. M., Mezzich, J., Cornelius, M. D., Fabreago, H., Ehler, J. G., Ulrich, R. F., Thase, M. E., & Mann, J. J. (1995). Disproportionate suicidality in patients with comorbid major depression and alcoholism. *American Journal of Psychiatry, 152,* 358–364.

Cornelius, J. R., Salloum, I. M., Thase, M. E., Haskett, R. F., Daley, D. C., Jones-Barlock, A., Pusher, C., & Perel, J. M. (1998). Fluoxetine versus placebo in depressed alcoholic cocaine abusers. *Psychopharmacology Bulletin, 34,* 117–121.

Corrigan, J. D., Lamb-Hart, G. L., & Rust, E. (1995). A programme of intervention for substance abuse following traumatic brain injury. *Brain Injury, 9,* 221–236.

Cox, G. B., Walker, R. D., Freng, S. A., Short, B. A., Meijer, L. & Gilchrist, L. (1998). Outcome of controlled trial of the effectiveness of intensive case management for chronic public inebriates. *Journal of Studies of Alcohol, 59,* 523–532.

Cramer, J., & Rosenheck, R. (1999). Enhancing medication compliance for people with serious mental illness. *Journal of Nervous and Mental Disease, 187,* 53–55.

Cuffel, B. J., Heithoff, K. A., & Lawson, W. (1993). Correlates of patterns of substance abuse among patients with schizophrenia. *Hospital and Community Psychiatry, 44,* 247–251.

Cui, X. J., & Vaillant, G. E. (1997). Does depression generate life events? *Journal of Nervous and Mental Disease, 185,* 145–150.

Cunningham, J. A., Sobell, L. C., Sobell, M. B., & Gaskin, J. (1994). Alcohol and drug abuser's reasons for seeking treatment. *Addictive Behaviors, 19,* 691–696.

Daley, D. D., & Zuckhoff, A. (1999). *Improving treatment compliance: Counseling and system strategies for substance abuse and dual disorders.* Center City, MN: Hazelden.

Daley, S. E., Hammen, C., Davila, J., & Burge, D. (1998). Axis II symptomatology, depression and life stress during the transition from adolescence to adulthood. *Journal of Consulting and Clinical Psychology, 66,* 595–603.

Davidson, J. R. (1997). Use of benzodiazepines in panic disorder. *Journal of Clinical Psychiatry, 58,* 26–28.

Davies, M. I., & Clark, D. M. (1998). Thought suppression produces a rebound effect with analogue post-traumatic intrusions. *Behaviour Research and Therapy*, *36*, 571–582.

Denton, R. E., & Kampfe, C. M. (1994). The relationship between family variables and adolescent substance abuse: A literature review. *Adolescence*, *29*, 475–495.

DeRubeis, R. J., & Crits-Christoph, P. (1998). Empirically supported individual and group treatments for adult mental disorders. *Journal of Consulting and Clinical Psychology*, *66*, 37–52.

DeRubeis, R. J., Gelfand, L. A., Tang, T. Z., & Simons, A. D. (1999). Medications versus cognitive behavior therapy for severely depressed outpatients: Meta-analysis of four randomized comparisons. *American Journal of Psychiatry*, *156*, 1007–1013.

Deykin, E. Y., & Buka, S. L. (1994). Suicidal ideation and attempts among chemically dependent adolescents. *American Journal of Public Health*, *84*, 634–639.

Dixon, L., McNary, S., & Lehman, A. (1997). One-year follow-up of secondary versus primary mental disorder in persons with comorbid substance use disorders. *American Journal of Psychiatry*, *154*, 1610–1612.

Dixon, L., McNary, S., & Lehman, A. F. (1998). Remission of substance use disorder among psychiatric inpatients with mental illness. *American Journal of Psychiatry*, *155*, 239–243.

Doering, S., Muller, E., Kopcke, W., Peitzcker, A., & Gaebael, W. (1998). Predictors of relapse and rehospitalization in schizophrenia and schizoaffective disorder. *Schizophrenia Bulletin*, *24*, 87–98.

Drake, R. E., & Mercer-McFadden, C. (1995). Assessment of substance use among persons with severe mental disorders. In A. F. Lehman & L. B. Dixon (Eds.), *Double jeopardy: Chronic mental illness and substance use disorders* (pp. 28–41). New York: Harwood Academic Press.

Drake, R. E., Mueser, K. T., Clark, R. E., & Wallach, M. A. (1996). The course, treatment and outcome of substance disorder in persons with severe mental illness. *American Journal of Orthopsychiatry*, *66*, 42–51.

Drake, R. E., Mueser, K. T., & McHugo, G. J. (1996). Clinician rating scales: Alcohol Use Scale (AUS), Drug Use Scale (DUS) and Substance Abuse Treatment Scale (SATS). In L. I. Sederer & E. Dickey (Eds.), *Outcomes assessment in clinical practice* (pp. 113–116). Baltimore, MD: Williams & Wilkins.

Drake, R. E., & Noordsy, D. L. (1994). Case management for people with co-existing severe mental disorder and substance use disorder. *Psychiatric Annals*, *24*, 427–431.

Drake, R. E., Rosenberg, S. D., & Mueser, K. T. (1996). Assessing substance use disorder in persons with severe mental illness. *New Directions for Mental Health Services*, *70*, 3–17.

Drake, R. E., & Wallach, M. A. (1993). Moderate drinking among people with severe mental illness. *Hospital and Community Psychiatry*, *44*, 780–782.

Drake, R. E., Yovetich, N. A., Bebout, R. B., Harris, M., & McHugo, G. J. (1997). Integrated treatment for dually diagnosed homeless adults. *Journal of Nervous and Mental Disease*, *185*, 298–305.

Duncan, S. C., Duncan, T. E., & Hops, H. (1998). Progressions of alcohol, cigarettes and marijuana use in adolescence. *Journal of Behavioral Medicine, 21,* 375–388.

Dutton, M. A., Burghardt, K. J., Perrin, S. G., Chrestman, K. R., & Halle, P. M. (1994). Battered women's cognitive schema. *Journal of Traumatic Stress, 7,* 237–255.

Egelko, S., & Galanter, M. (1998). Impact of social anxiety in a "therapeutic community"-oriented cocaine treatment clinic. *American Journal of Addiction, 7,* 136–141.

el-Guebaly, N., & Hodgins, D. C. (1992). Schizophrenia and substance abuse: Prevalence issues. *Canadian Journal of Psychiatry, 37,* 704–710.

Elliott, R., Sahakian, B. J., McKay, A. T., Robbins, T. W., & Paykel, E. S. (1996). Neuropsychological impairments in unipolar depression: The influence of perceived failure on subsequent performance. *Psychological Medicine, 26,* 975–989.

Epstein, E. E., Ginsburg, B. E., Hesselbrock, V. M., & Schwarz, J. C. (1994). Alcohol and drug abusers subtyped by antisocial personality and primary or secondary depressive disorder. *Annals of the New York Academy of Science, 708,* 187–201.

Erickson, D. H., Beiser, M., & Iacono, W. G. (1998). Social support predicts 5-year outcome in first-episode schizophrenia. *Journal of Abnormal Psychology, 107,* 681–685.

Evans, K. (1999). *The conversion experience: A phenomenological study of the addicted adolescent female survivor and her motivation to change* (dissertation). Minneapolis: Graduate School of America.

Evans, K., & Sullivan, J. M. (1995). *Treating addicted survivors of trauma.* New York: Guilford Press.

Fanco, H. (1995). Combining behavioral and self-help approaches in the inpatient management of dually diagnosed patients. *Journal of Substance Abuse Treatment, 12,* 227–232.

Fein, G., Bachman, L., Fisher, S., & Davenport, L. (1990). Cognitive impairments in abstinent alcoholics. *Western Journal of Medicine, 152,* 531–537.

Feinman, J. A., & Dunner, D. L. (1996). The effect of alcohol and substance abuse on the course of bipolar affective disorder. *Journal of Affective Disorders, 37,* 43–49.

Felton, J. S. (1998). Burnout as a clinical entity—its importance in health care workers. *Occupational Medicine, 48,* 237–250.

Fenton, W. S., Blyler, C. R., & Heinssen, R. K. (1997). Determinants of medication compliance in schizophrenia: Empirical and clinical findings. *Schizophrenia Bulletin, 23,* 637–651.

Figueroa, E. F., Silk, K. R., Huth, A., & Lohr, N. E. (1997). History of childhood sexual abuse and general psychopathology. *Comprehensive Psychiatry, 38,* 23–30.

Finney, J. W., Noyes, C. A., Coutts, A. I., & Moos, R. H. (1998). Evaluating substance abuse treatment process models: I. Changes on proximal outcome variables during 12-step and cognitive-behavioral treatment. *Journal of Studies of Alcohol, 59,* 371–380.

Flaum, M., & Schultz, S. K. (1996). When does amphetamine-induced psychosis become schizophrenia? *American Journal of Psychiatry, 153,* 812–815.

Fleisch, B. (1991). *Approaches in the treatment of adolescents with emotional and substance abuse problems.* (DHHS Publication No. [SMA] 93–1744). Rockville, MD: Center for Substance Abuse Treatment, Substance Abuse and Mental Health Services Administration, Public Health Service, U.S. Department of Health and Human Services.

Foa, B. E., Rothbaum, B. O., Riggs, D. S., & Murdock, T. B. (1991). Treatment of post-traumatic stress disorder in rape victims: A comparison between cognitive-behavioral procedures and counseling. *Journal of Consulting and Clinical Psychology, 59,* 715–723.

Forehand, R., Miller, K. S., Dutra, R., & Chance, M. W. (1997). Role of parenting in adolescent deviant behavior: Replication across and within two ethnic groups. *Journal of Consulting and Clinical Psychology, 65,* 1036–1041.

Gacono, C. B., Meloy, J. R., & Berg, J. L. (1992). Object relations, defensive operations and affective states in narcissistic, borderline and antisocial personality disorder. *Journal of Personality Assessment, 59,* 32–49.

Galanter, M. (1993). *Network therapy for alcohol and drug abuse: A new approach in practice.* New York: Basic Books.

Galvin, M., Shekhar, A., Simon, J., Stillwell, B., Ten Eyck, R., Laite, G., Karwisch, G., & Blix, G. (1991). Low dopamine-beta hydroxylase: A biological sequela of abuse and neglect? *Psychiatry Research, 39,* 1–11.

Geller, A. (1998). Neurological effects. In A. W. Graham, T. K. Schultz, & B. B. Wilford (Eds.), *Principles of addiction medicine* (pp. 775–792). Chevy Chase, MD: American Society of Addiction Medicine.

Gibson, D. R., Sorensen, J. L., Wermuth, L., & Bernal, G. (1992). Families are helped by drug treatment. *International Journal of Addictions, 27,* 961–978.

Gillen, R., & Hesselbrock, V. (1992). Cognitive functioning, ASP and family history of alcoholism in young men at risk for alcoholism. *Alcohol: Clinical and Experimental Research, 16,* 206–214.

Goldberg, S. C., Schooler, N. R., Hogarty, G. E., & Roper, M. (1977). Prediction of relapse in schizophrenic patients treated by drug and social therapy. *Archives of General Psychiatry, 34,* 171–184.

Goldman, M. S. (1990). Experience-dependent neuropsychological recovery and the treatment of chronic alcoholism. *Neuropsychology Review, 1,* 75–101.

Gorey, K. M., Leslie, D. R., Morris, T., Carruthers, W. V., John, L., & Chacko, J. (1998). Effectiveness of case management with severely and persistently mentally ill people. *Community Mental Health Journal, 34,* 241–250.

Gorski, T. T. (1989). *Passages through recovery: An action plan for preventing relapse.* New York: Harper & Row.

Gortner, E. T., Gollan, J. K., Dobson, K. S., & Jacobson, N. S. (1998). Cognitive-behavioral treatment for depression: Relapse prevention. *Journal of Consulting and Clinical Psychology, 66,* 377–384.

Gotham, H. J., & Sher, K. J. (1996). Children of alcoholics. In J. Kinney (Ed.), *Clinical manual of substance abuse* (2nd ed., pp. 272–300). St. Louis, MO: Mosby Year Book.

Grant, B. F. (1995). Comorbidity between DSM-IV drug use disorders and major depression: Results of a national survey of adults. *Journal of Substance Abuse, 74,* 481–497.

Grant, B. F., Hasin, D. S., & Dawson, D. A. (1996). The relationship between DSM-IV alcohol use disorders and DSM-IV major depression: Examination of the primary–secondary distinction in a general population sample. *Journal of Affective Disorders, 38*, 113–128.

Grant, B. F., & Pickering, R. P. (1996). Comorbidity between DSM-IV alcohol and drug use disorders: Results from the National Longitudinal Alcohol Epidemiological Survey. *Alcohol Health and Research World, 20*, 67–75.

Greene, R. L., Weed, N. C., Butcher, J. N., Arredondo, R., & Davis, H. G. (1992). A cross-validation of MMPI-2 substance abuse scales. *Journal of Personality Assessment, 58*, 5–10.

Greenfield, S. F., Weiss, R. D., Muenz, L. R., Vagge, L. M., Kelly, J. F., Bello, L. R., & Michael, J. (1998). The effect of depression on return to drinking: A prospective study. *Archives of General Psychiatry, 55*, 259–265.

Grillon, Dierker, L., & Merikangas, K. R. (1997). Startle modulation in children at risk for anxiety disorders and/or alcoholism. *Journal of the American Academy of Child and Adolescent Psychiatry, 36*, 925–932.

Grilo, C. M., Becker, D. F., Fehon, D. C., Edell, W. S. & McGlashan, T. H. (1996). Conduct disorder, substance use disorders and coexisting conduct and substance use disorders in adolescent inpatients. *American Journal of Psychiatry, 153*, 914–920.

Grilo, C. M., Becker, D. F., Walker, M. L., Levy, K. N., Edell, W. S., & McGlashan, T. H. (1995). Psychiatric co-morbidity in adolescent inpatients with substance use disorders. *Journal of the American Academy of Child and Adolescent Psychiatry, 34*, 1085–1091.

Grove, W. M., Eckert, E. D., Heston, L., Bouchard, T. J., Segal, N. & Lykken, D. T. (1990). Heritability of substance abuse and antisocial behavior: A study of monzygotic twins reared apart. *Biological Psychiatry, 27*, 1293–1304.

Gunderson, J. G. (1996). The borderline patient's intolerance of aloneness: Insecure attachments and therapist availability. *American Journal of Psychiatry, 153*, 752–758.

Gunderson, J. G., Frank, A. F., Katz, H. M., Vannicell, I. T., Frosch, J. P., & Knapp, P. H. (1994). Effects of psychotherapy in schizophrenia: II. Comparative outcome of two forms of treatment. *Schizophrenia Bulletin, 10*, 564–598.

Gupchup, G. V., Lively, B. T., Holiday-Goodman, M., Siganga, W. W., & Black, C. D. (1994). Maslach Burnout Inventory: Factor structures for pharmacists in health maintenance organizations and comparison with normative data for USA pharmacists. *Psychology Reports, 74*, 891–895.

Harvey, A. G., & Bryant, R. A. (1998). The effect of attempted thought suppression in acute stress disorder. *Behaviour Research and Therapy, 36*, 583–590.

Hastings-Vertino, K. A. (1996). STEMSS (Support Together for Mental and Emotional Serenity and Sobriety): An alternative to traditional forms of self-help for the dually diagnosed consumer. *Journal of Addictions Nursing, 8*, 20–28.

Haywood, T. W., Kravitz, H. M., Grossman, L. S., Cavanaugh, J. L., Davis, J. M. & Lewis, D. A. (1995). Predicting the "Revolving Door" phenomenon among patients with schizophrenic, schizoaffective and affective disorders. *American Journal of Psychiatry, 152,* 856–861.

Hellerstein, D. J., & Meehan, B. (1987). Outpatient group therapy for schizophrenic substance abusers. *American Journal of Psychiatry, 144,* 1337–1339.

Henggeler, S. W., Pickrel, S. G., Brondino, M. J., & Crouch, J. L. (1996). Eliminating (almost) treatment dropout of substance abusing or dependent delinquents through home-based multisystemic therapy. *American Journal of Psychiatry, 153,* 427–428.

Hernandez, J. T. (1992). Substance abuse among sexually abused adolescents and their families. *Journal of Adolescent Health, 13,* 658–662.

Hesselbrock, M. N., Meyer, R. E., & Keener, J. J. (1985). Psychopathology in hospitalized alcoholics. *Archives of General Psychiatry, 42,* 1050–1055.

Higgins, S. T., Delaney, D. D., Budney, A. J., Bickel, W. K., Hughes, J. R., Foerg, F., & Fenwick, J. W. (1991). A behavioral approach to achieving initial abstinence. *American Journal of Psychiatry, 148,* 1218–1224.

Hoffmann, J. P. (1995). The effects of family structure and family relationships on adolescent marijuana use. *International Journal of Addiction, 30,* 1207–1241.

Hogarty, G. E., Kornblith, S. J., Greenwald, D., Dibarry, A. L., Colley, S., Ulrich, R. F., Carter, M., & Flesher, S. (1997). Three-year trials of personal therapy among schizophrenic patients living with or independent of family: I. Description of study and effects on relapse rates. *American Journal of Psychiatry, 154,* 1504–1513.

Holland, R., Moretti, M. M., Verlan, V., & Peterson, S. (1993). Attachment and conduct disorder: The Response Program. *Canadian Journal of Psychiatry, 38,* 420–431.

Honig, A., Hofman, A., Rozendaal, N., & Dingemanns, P. (1997). Psychoeducation in bipolar disorder: Effect on expressed emotion. *Psychiatry Research, 72,* 17–22.

Hudziak, J. J., Boffeli, T. J., Kriesman, J. J., Battaglia, M. M., Stanger, C., & Guze, S. B. (1996). Clinical study of the relations of borderline personality disorder to Briquet's syndrome (hysteria), somatization disorder, antisocial personality disorder and substance abuse disorders. *American Journal of Psychiatry, 153,* 1598–1606.

Humes, D. L., & Humphrey, L. L. (1994). A multi-method analysis of families with a poly-drug dependent or normal adolescent daughter. *Journal of Abnormal Psychology, 103,* 676–685.

Hunt, G. M., & Azrin, N. H. (1973). A community-reinforcement approach to alcoholism. *Behaviour Research and Therapy, 11,* 91–104.

Iguchi, M. Y., Lamb, R. J., Belding, M. A., Platt, J. J., Husband, S. D., & Morral, A. R. (1996). Contingent reinforcement of group participation versus abstinence in a methadone maintenance program. *Experimental and Clinical Psychopharmacology, 4,* 315–321.

Isenhart, C. E., & Silversmith, D. J. (1996). MMPI-2 response styles: Generalization to alcoholism assessment. *Psychology of Addictive Behaviors, 10,* 115–123.

Jackson, C. A., Manning, W. G., Jr., & Wells, K. B. (1995). Impact of prior and current alcohol use on use of services by patients with depression and chronic medical illnesses. *Health Services Research, 30,* 687–705.

Jaffe, A. J., Rounsaville, B., Chang, G., Schottenfeld, R. S., Meyer, R. E. & O'Malley, S. S. (1996). Naltrexone, relapse prevention and supportive therapy with alcoholics: An analysis of patient treatment matching. *Journal of Consulting and Clinical Psychology, 64,* 1044–1053.

Jefferson, J. W. (1997). Antidepressants in panic disorder. *Journal of Clinical Psychiatry, 64,* 20–24.

Jerrell, J. M., & Ridgely, M. S. (1995). Comparative effectiveness of three approaches to serving people with severe mental illness and substance abuse disorders. *Journal of Nervous and Mental Disease, 183,* 566–576.

Johnson, M. R., & Lydiard, R. B. (1995). The neurobiology of anxiety disorders. *Psychiatric Clinics of North America, 18,* 681–725.

Johnson, R. J., & Kaplan, H. B. (1990). Stability of psychological symptoms: Drug use consequences and intervening processes. *Journal of Health and Social Behavior, 31,* 277–291.

Johnson, S. L., & Miller, I. (1997). Negative life events and time to recovery from episodes of bipolar disorder. *Journal of Abnormal Psychology, 106,* 449–457.

Kadden, R., Carroll, K., Donovan, D., Cooney, N., Monti, P., Abrams, D., Litt, M., & Hester, R. (1994). *Cognitive-behavioral coping skills therapy manual: A clinical guide for therapists treating individuals with alcohol abuse and dependence* (Project Match Monograph Series, Vol. 3). Rockville, MD: U.S. Department of Health and Human Services, Public Health Service, National Institutes of Health, National Institute on Alcohol Abuse and Alcoholism.

Kahn, E. M., & Kahn, E. W. (1992). Group treatment assignment for outpatients with schizophrenia: Integrating recent clinical and research findings. *Community Mental Health Journal, 28,* 539–550.

Kessler, R. C. (1997). The effects of stressful life events on depression. *Annual Review of Psychology, 48,* 191–214.

Kessler, R. C., Crum, R. M., Warner, L. A., Nelson, C. B., Schulenber, J., & Anthony, J. C. (1997). Lifetime co-occurrence of DSM-II-R alcohol abuse and dependence with other psychiatric disorders in the National Comorbidity Survey. *Archives of General Psychiatry, 54,* 313–321.

Khantzian, E. J. (1997). The self-medication hypothesis of substance use disorders: A reconsideration and recent applications. *Harvard Review of Psychiatry, 4,* 231–244.

King, C. A., Ghaziuddin, N., McGovern, L., Brand, E., Hill, E., & Naylor, M. (1996). Predictors of comorbid alcohol and substance abuse in depressed adolescents. *Journal of the American Academy of Child and Adolescent Psychiatry, 35,* 743–751.

Kinney, J. (Ed.). (1996). *Clinical manual of substance abuse* (2nd ed.). St. Louis, MO: Mosby Year Book.

Kinney, J., & West, D. (1996). Substance use treatment. In J. Kinney (Ed.), *Clinical manual of substance abuse* (2nd ed., pp. 74–98). St. Louis, MO: Mosby Year Book.

Klingeman, J. K.-H. (1991). The motivation for change from problem alcohol and heroin use. *British Journal of Addiction, 86,* 727–744.

Kofoed, L., Kania, J., Walsh, T., & Atkinson, R. M. (1986). Outpatient treatment of patients with substance abuse and co-existing psychiatric disorders. *American Journal of Psychiatry, 143,* 867–872.

Kramer, T. H., & Hoisington, D. (1992). Use of AA and NA in the treatment of chemical dependencies of traumatic brain injury survivors. *Brain Injury, 6,* 81–88.

Krampen, G. (1989). Motivation in the treatment of alcoholism. *Addictive Behaviors, 14,* 197–200.

Kranzler, H. R. (1996). Evaluation and treatment of anxiety symptoms and disorders in alcoholics. *Journal of Clinical Psychiatry, 57,* 15–21.

Kranzler, H. R., & Liebowitz, N. R. (1988). Anxiety and depression in substance abuse. *Medical Clinics of North America, 72,* 867–885.

Kupfer, D. J. & Frank, E. (1997). Role of psychosocial factors in the onset of major depression. *Annals of the New York Academy of Sciences, 806,* 429–439.

Kurtz, E., & Ketchem, K. (1996). *The spirituality of imperfection.* New York: Bantam Books.

Kutcher, S. (1997). Practitioner review: The pharmacotherapy of adolescent depression. *Journal of Child Psychology and Psychiatry, 38,* 755–767.

Lauer, L., Black, D. W., & Keen, P. (1993). Multiple personality disorder and borderline personality disorder. Distinct entities or variations on a common theme? *Annals of Clinical Psychiatry, 5,* 129–134.

Lazowski, L. E., Miller, F. G., Boye, M. W., & Miller, G. M. (1998). Efficacy of the Substance Abuse Subtle Screening Inventory-3 (SASSI-3) in identifying substance dependence disorders in clinical settings. *Journal of Personality Assessment, 71,* 114–128.

Leal, J., Ziedonis, D., & Kosten, T. (1994). Antisocial personality disorder as a prognostic factor for pharmacotherapy of cocaine dependence. *Drug and Alcohol Dependence, 35,* 31–35.

LeDoux, J. (1996). *The emotional brain: The mysterious underpinnings of emotional life.* New York: Simon & Schuster.

Lehman, A. F. (1996). Heterogeneity of person and place: Assessing co-occurring addictive and mental disorders. *American Journal of Orthopsychiatry, 66,* 32–41.

Lehman, A. F., Myers, P. C., Dixon, L. B., & Johnson, J. L. (1996). Detection of substance use disorders among psychiatric inpatients. *The Journal of Nervous and Mental Disease, 184,* 228–233.

Leonard, K. E., & Roberts, L. J. (1998). The effects of alcohol on the marital interactions of aggressive and nonaggressive husbands and their wives. *Journal of Abnormal Psychology, 107,* 602–615.

Leshner, A. I. (1997). Addiction is a brain disease, and it matters. *Science, 278,* 45–47.

Levy, M. (1993). Psychotherapy with dual diagnosis patients: Working with denial. *Journal of Substance Abuse Treatment, 10,* 499–504.

Lewinsohn, P. M., Gotlib, I. H., & Seeley, J. R. (1995). Adolescent psychopathology: IV. Specificity of psychosocial risk factors for depression and substance abuse in older adolescents. *Journal of the American Academy of Child and Adolescent Psychiatry, 34*, 1221–1229.

Liberman, R. P., & Corrigan, P. W. (1993). Designing new psychosocial treatments for schizophrenia. *Psychiatry, 56*, 238–249.

Liberman, R. P., & Kopelowicz, A. (1995). Basic elements in biobehavioral treatment and rehabilitation of schizophrenia. *International Clinical Psychopharmacology, 9*, 51–58.

Liepman, M. R. (1993). Using family influence to motivate alcoholics to enter treatment: The Johnson Institute Intervention Approach. In T. J. O'Farrell (Ed.), *Treating alcohol problems: Marital and family interventions* (pp. 54–77). New York: Guilford Press.

Lin, N., Eisen, S. A., Scherrer, J. F., Goldberg, J., True, W. R., Lyons, M. J., & Tsuang, M. T. (1996). The influence of familial and non-familial factors on the association between major depression and substance abuse/dependence in 1874 monozygotic male twin pairs. *Drug and Alcohol Dependence, 43*, 49–55.

Linehan, M. M. (1993). *Cognitive-behavioral treatment of borderline personality disorder*. New York: Guilford Press.

Links, P. S., Helgrave, R. J., Mitton, J. E., van Reekum, R., & Patrick, J. (1995). Borderline personality disorder and substance abuse: Consequences of comorbidity. *Canadian Journal of Psychiatry, 40*, 9–14.

Links, P. S. & van Reekum, R. (1993). Childhood sexual abuse, parental impairment and the development of borderline personality disorder. *Canadian Journal of Psychiatry, 38*, 472–474.

Loeber, R. & Strouthamer-Loeber, M. (1998). Development of juvenile aggression and violence: Some common misconceptions and controversies. *American Psychologist, 53*, 242–259.

Longabaugh, R., Beattie, M., Noel, S., Stout, R., & Malloy, P. (1993). The effect of social investment on treatment outcome. *Journal of Studies on Alcohol, 54*, 465–478.

Longabaugh, R., Wirtz, P. W., Zweben, A., & Stout, R. L. (1998). Network support for drinking, Alcoholics Anonymous and long-term matching effects. *Addiction, 93*, 1313–1333.

Lydiard, R. B., Brawman-Mintzer, O., & Ballenger, J. C. (1996). Recent developments in the psychopharmacology of anxiety disorders. *Journal of Consulting and Clinical Psychology, 64*, 660–668.

Lyons, J. S., & McGovern, M. P. (1989). Use of mental health services by dually diagnosed patients. *Hospital and Community Psychiatry, 40*, 1067–1069.

Lyons, M. J., True, W. R., Eisen, S. A., Goldberg, J., Meyer, J., Faraone, S. V., Eaves, L. J., & Tsuang, M. T. (1995). Differential heritability of adult and juvenile antisocial traits. *Archives of General Psychiatry, 52*, 906–915.

MacPherson, R., Jerrom, B., & Hughes, A. (1996). A controlled study of education about drug treatment in schizophrenia. *British Journal of Psychiatry, 168*, 709–717.

Maisto, S. A., McKay, J. R., & Connors, G. J. (1990). Self-report issues in substance abuse: State of the art and future directions. *Behavioral Assessment,*
12, 117–134.

Margolis, R. D., & Zweben, J. (1998). *Treating patients with alcohol and other drug*
problems: An integrated approach. Washington, DC: American Psychological
Association.

Mason, B. J., Kocsis, J. H., Ritvo, E. C., & Cutler, R. B. (1996). A double-blind
placebo-controlled trials of desipramine in primary alcoholics stratified on
the presence or absence of major depression. *Journal of the American Medi-*
cal Association, 275, 1–7.

McCrady, B. S. (1994). Alcoholics Anonymous and behavior therapy: Can habits be treated as diseases? Can diseases be treated as habits? *Journal of Con-*
sulting and Clinical Psychology, 62, 1159–1166.

McCrady, B. S., & Epstein, E. E. (1996). Theoretical bases of family approaches
to substance abuse treatment. In F. Rotgers, D. S. Keller, & J. Morgernstern
(Eds.), *Treating substance abuse: Theory and technique* (pp. 117–142). New
York: Guilford Press.

McGlashan, T. H., & Fenton, W. S. (1992). The positive-negative distinction in
schizophrenia: Review of natural history validators. *Archives of General Psy-*
chiatry, 49, 63–72.

McGrath, P. J., Nunes, E. V., Stewart, J. W., Goldman, D., Agosti, V., Ocepek-
Welikson, K., & Quitkin, F. M. (1996). Imipramine treatment of alcoholics
with primary depression: A placebo-controlled clinical trial. *Archives of*
General Psychiatry, 53, 232–240.

McKay, J. R., Alterman, A. I., Cassiola, J. S., Rutherford, M. J., O'Brien, C. P., &
Koppenhaver, J. (1997). Group counseling versus individualized relapse
prevention aftercare following intensive outpatient treatment for cocaine
dependence: Initial results. *Journal of Consulting and Clinical Psychology, 65,*
778–788.

McKnight, J. D., & Glass, D. C. (1995). Perceptions of control, burnout, and
depressive symptomatology: A replication and extension. *Journal of Con-*
sulting and Clinical Psychology, 63, 490–494.

McLellan, A. T., Alterman, A. I., Metzger, D. S., Grissom, G. R., Woody, G. E.,
Luborsky, L. & O'Brien, C.P. (1994). Similarity of outcome predictors
across opiate, cocaine, and alcohol treatments: Role of treatment services.
Journal of Consulting and Clinical Psychology, 62, 1141–1158.

McLellan, A. T., Grissom, G. R., Zanis, D., Randall, M., Brill, P., & O'Brien, C. P,
(1997). Problems-service "matching" in addiction treatment: A prospective study in 4 programs. *Archives of General Psychiatry, 54,* 730–735.

Meehan, W., O'Connor, L. E., Berry, J. W., Weiss, J., Morrison, A., & Acampora,
A. (1996). Guilt, shame and depression in clients in recovery from addiction. *Journal of Psychoactive Drugs, 28,* 125–134.

Mee-Lee, D. (1994). Managed care and dual diagnosis. In N. S. Miller (Ed.),
Treating coexisting Psychiatric and addictive disorders: A practical guide (pp. 257–
269). Center City, MN: Hazelden.

Meichenbaum, D. (1994). *A clinical handbook/practical therapist manual for assess-*

ing and treating adults with post-traumatic stress disorder (PTSD). Waterloo, Ontario, Canada: Institute Press.

Meltzer, H. Y. (1993). New drugs for the treatment of schizophrenia. *Psychiatric Clinics of North America, 16*, 365–385.

Milberger, S., Biederman, J., Faraone, S. V., Murphy, J., & Tsuang, T. (1995). Attention Deficit Hyperactivity Disorder and comorbid disorders: Issues of overlapping symptoms. *American Journal of Psychiatry, 152*, 1793–1799.

Miller, N. S., & Chappell, J. N. (1991). History of the disease concept. *Psychiatric Annals, 21*, 196–205.

Miller, W. R., Benefield, R. G., & Tonigan, J. S. (1993). Enhancing motivation for change in problem drinking: A controlled comparison of two therapist styles. *Journal of Consulting and Clinical Psychology, 61*, 455–461.

Miller, W. R., Brown, J. M., Simpson, T. L., Handmaker, N. S., Bien, T. H., Luckie, L. F., Montgomery, H. A., Hester, R. K., & Tonigan, J. S. (1995). What works?: A methodological analysis of the alcohol treatment outcome literature. In R. K. Hester & W. R. Miller (Eds.), *Handbook of alcoholism treatment approaches: Effective alternatives* (2nd ed.). Boston: Allyn & Bacon.

Miller, W. R., Meyers, R. J., & Tonigan, J. S. (1999). Engaging the unmotivated in treatment for alcohol problems: A comparison of three strategies for intervention through family members. *Journal of Consulting and Clinical Psychology, 67*, 688–697.

Miller, W. R., & Rollnick, S. (1991). *Motivational interviewing: Preparing people to change addictive behavior*. New York: Guilford Press.

Miller, W. R., Zweben, A., DiClemente, C. C., & Rychtarik, R. G. (1994). *Motivational enhancement therapy manual* (NIAAA Project Match Monograph Series No. 2, NIH Pub. No. 94–3723). Rockville, MD: U.S. Department of Health and Human Services.

Miller-Johnson, S., Lochman, J. E., Coie, J. D., Terry, R., & Hyman, C. (1998). Comorbidity of conduct and depressive problems at sixth grade: Substance use outcomes across adolescence. *Journal of Abnormal Child Psychology, 26*, 221–232.

Minkoff, K., & Rossi, A. (1998). *Report of the Center for Mental Health Services Managed Care Initiative: Clinical Standards and Workforce Competencies Project, Co-Occuring Mental and Substance Disorders Panel*. Philadelphia: Center for Mental Health Policy and Services Research, Department of Psychiatry and Substance Abuse and Mental Health Services Administration, University of Pennsylvania Health System.

Molly, D. (1992). Dual diagnosis and the ASAM placement criteria. *The Counselor*, 14–17.

Monti, P. M., Abrams, D. B., Kadden, R. H., & Cooney, N. L. (1989). *Treating alcohol dependence: A coping skills training guide*. New York: Guilford Press.

Morgenstern, J., Labouvie, E., McCrady, B. S., Kahler, C. W., & Frey, R. M. (1997). Affiliation with Alcoholics Anonymous: A study of its therapeutic effects and mechanisms of action. *Journal of Consulting and Clinical Psychology, 65*, 768–777.

Mueller, T. I., Lavori, P. W., Keller, M. B., Swartz, A., Warshaw, M., Hasin, D., Coryell, W., Endicott, J., Rice, J., & Akiskal, H. (1994). Prognostic effect of the variable course of alcoholism on the 10-year course of depression. *American Journal of Psychiatry, 151,* 701–706.

Mueser, K. T., Bellack, A. S., & Blanchard, J. J. (1992). Comorbidity of schizophrenia and substance abuse: Implications for treatment. *Journal of Consulting and Clinical Psychology, 60,* 845–856.

Najavits, L. M, Griffin, M., Luborsky, L., & Frank, A. (1995). Therapists' emotional reactions to substance abusers: A new questionnaire and initial findings. *Psychotherapy, 32,* 669–677.

Newcomb, M. D., Scheier, L. M. & Bentler, P.M. (1993). Effects of adolescent drug use on adult mental health: A prospective study of a community sample. *Experimental and Clinical Psychopharmacology, 1,* 215–241.

Newman, J. P., Kosson, D. S., & Patterson, C. M. (1992). Delay of gratification in psychopathic and nonpsychopathic offenders. *Journal of Abnormal Psychology, 101,* 630–636.

Nixon, S. J., & Glenn, S. W. (1995). Cognitive psychosocial performance and recovery in female alcoholics. *Recent Developments in Alcoholism, 12,* 287–307.

Norman, R. M., & Malla, A. K. (1993). Stressful life events and schizophrenia: I. A review of the research. *British Journal of Psychiatry, 162,* 161–166.

O'Brien, C.P. (1996). Recent developments in the pharmacotherapy of substance abuse. *Journal of Consulting and Clinical Psychology, 64,* 677–686.

O'Connor, P. G. (1996). Routine screening and initial assessment. In J. Kinney (Ed.), *Clinical manual of substance abuse,* (2nd ed., pp. 40–73). St. Louis, MO: Mosby Year Book.

O'Farrell, T. J. (1993). A behavioral marital therapy couples group program for alcoholics and their spouses. In T. J. O'Farrell (Ed.), *Treating alcohol problems: Marital and family interventions* (pp. 170–209). New York: Guilford Press.

O'Farrell, T. J., Hooley, J., Fals-Stewart, W., & Cutter, H. S. G. (1998). Expressed emotion and relapse in alcoholic patients. *Journal of Consulting and Clinical Psychology, 66,* 744–752.

Oldham, J. M., Skodol, A. E., Gallaher, P. E., & Kroll, M. E. (1996). Relationship of borderline symptoms to histories of abuse and neglect: A pilot study. *Psychiatric Quarterly, 67,* 287–295.

Osher, F. C. (1996). Dual diagnosis. In J. Kinney (Ed.), *Clinical manual of substance abuse* (2nd ed., pp. 245–253). St. Louis, MO: Mosby Year Book.

Osher, F. C., & Drake, R. E. (1996). Reversing a history of unmet needs: Approaches to care for persons with co-occurring addictive and mental disorders. *American Journal of Orthopsychiatry, 66,* 4–11.

Osher, F. C., & Kofoed, L. L. (1989).Treatment of patients with psychiatric and psychoactive substance abuse disorders. *Hospital and Community Psychiatry, 40,* 1025–1030.

Otto, R. K., Long, A. R., Megaree, E. I., & Rosenblatt, A. I. (1988). Ability of alcoholics to escape detection by the MMPI. *Journal of Consulting and Clinical Psychology, 56,* 452–457.

Ouimette, P. C., Finney, J. W., & Moos, R. H. (1997). Twelve-Step and cognitive-behavioral treatment for substance abuse: A comparison of treatment effectiveness. (1997). *Journal of Consulting and Clinical Psychology, 65,* 230–240.

Owen, R. R., Fischer, E. P., Booth, B. M., & Cuffel, B. J. (1996). Medication noncompliance and substance abuse among patients with schizophrenia. *Psychiatric Services, 47,* 853–858.

Parikh, S. V., Kusumakar, V., Haslam, D. R., Matte, R., Sharma, V., & Yatham, L. N. (1997). Psychosocial interventions as an adjunct to pharmacotherapy in bipolar disorder. *Canadian Journal of Psychiatry, 42,* 74S–78S.

Paris, J. (1996). Antisocial personality disorder: A biopsychosocial model. *Canadian Journal of Psychiatry, 41,* 75–80.

Parsons, O. A. (1998). Neurocognitive deficits in alcoholics and social drinkers: A continuum? *Alcohol: Clinical and Experimental Research, 22,* 954–961.

Patterson, G. R., Reid, J. B., & Dishion, T. J. (1992). *A social interfactional approach: IV. Antisocial boys.* Eugene, OR: Castalia.

Penick, E. C., Powell, B. J., Campbell, J., Liskow, B. I., Nickel, E. J., Dale, T. M., Thomas, H. M., Laster, L. J., & Noble, E. (1996). Pharmacological treatment for antisocial personality disorder alcoholics: A preliminary study. *Alcohol: Clinical and Experimental Research, 20,* 477–484.

Penick, E. C., Powell, B. J., Liskow, B. I., Jackson, J. O., & Nickel, E. J. (1984). The stability of existing psychiatric syndromes in alcoholic men after one year. *Journal of Studies on Alcohol, 49,* 395–405.

Perry, A., Tarrier, N., Morriss, R., McCarthy, E., & Limb, K. (1999). Randomized controlled trial of efficacy of teaching patients with bipolar disorder to identify early symptoms of relapse and obtain treatment. *British Medical Journal, 318,* 149–153.

Pliszka, S. R., Carlson, C. L., & Swanson, J. M. (1999). *ADHD with comorbid disorders: Clinical assessment and management.* New York: Guilford Press.

Pope, H. G., Jr., Gruber, A. J., & Yurgelun-Todd, D. (1995). The residual neuropsychological effects of cannabis: The current status of research. *Drug and Alcohol Dependence, 38,* 25–34.

Post, R. M. (1990). Non-lithium treatment for bipolar disorder. *Journal of Clinical Psychiatry, 51 (Suppl. 8),* 9–16.

Prince, S. E., & Jacobson, N. S. (1995). A review and evaluation of marital and family therapies for affective disorders. *Journal of Marital and Family Therapy, 21,* 377–401.

Prochaska, J. O., DiClemente, C. C., & Norcross, J. C. In search of how people change: Applications to addictive behaviors. (1992). *American Psychologist, 47,* 1102–1114.

Project Match Research Group. (1997). Matching alcoholism treatments to client heterogeneity: Project MATCH posttreatment drinking outcomes. *Journal of Studies on Alcohol, 58,* 7–29.

Purcell, R., Maruff, P., Kyrios, M., & Pantelis, C. (1998). Neuropsychological deficits in obsessive-compulsive disorder: A comparison with unipolar depression, panic disorder and normal controls. *Archives of General Psychiatry, 55,* 415–423.

Reed, R. J., Grant, I., & Rourke, S. B. (1992). Long-term abstinent alcoholics have normal memory. *Alcohol: Clinical and Experimental Research, 16,* 677–683.

Regier, D. A., Farmer, M. E., Rae, D. S., Locke, B. Z., Keith, S. J., Judd, L. J., & Goodwin, F. K. (1990). Comorbidity of mental disorders with alcohol and other drug abuse: Results from the Epidemiologic Catchment Area (ECA) Study. *Journal of the American Medical Association, 264,* 2511–2518.

Reynolds, C. F., 3rd, Frank, E., Perel, J. M., Imber, S. D., Cornes, C., Miller, M. D., Mazumdar, S., Houck, P. R., Dew, M. A., Stack, J. A., Pollock, B. G., & Kupfer, D. J. (1999). Nortriptyline and interpersonal psychotherapy as maintenance therapies for recurring depression: A randomized controlled trial in patients older than 59 years. *Journal of the American Medical Association, 281,* 83–84.

Ries, R. K., & Miller, N. S. (1993). Dual diagnosis: Concept, diagnosis and treatment. In D. L. Dunner (Ed.), *Current psychiatric therapy* (pp. 131–138). Philadelphia, PA: Saunders.

Robinson, D., Woerner, M. G., Alvir, J. M., Bilder, R., Goldman, R., Geisler, S., Koreen, A., Sheitman, B., Chakos, M., Mayerhoff, D., & Lieberman, J. A. (1999). Predictors of relapse from a first episode of schizophrenia or schizoaffective disorder. *Archives of General Psychiatry, 56,* 241–247.

Rosenbaum, J. F., Pollack, M. H., & Pollack, R. A. (1996). Clinical Issues in the long-term treatment of panic disorder. *Journal of Clinical Psychiatry, 57,* 44–48.

Rosenbaum, M., Lewinsohn, P. M., & Gotlib, I. H. (1996). Distinguishing between state-dependent and non-state-dependent depression-related psychosocial variables. *British Journal of Clinical Psychology, 35,* 341–358.

Rosenberg, H. (1993). Prediction of controlled drinking by alcoholics and problem drinkers. *Psychological Bulletin, 113,* 129–139.

Rosenheck, R. (1995). Substance abuse and the chronically mentally ill: Therapeutic alliance and therapeutic limit-setting. *Community Mental Health Journal, 31,* 283–285.

Rosenheck, R., Dunn, L., Peszke, M., Cramer, J., Xu, W., Thomas, J., & Charney, D. (1999). Impact of clozapine on negative symptoms and on the deficit syndrome in refractory schizophrenia. Department of Veterans Affairs Cooperative Study Group on Clozapine in Refractory Schizophrenia. *American Journal of Psychiatry, 156,* 88–93.

Rounsaville, B. J., Dolinsky, Z. S., Babor, T. F., & Meyer, R. E. (1987). Psychopathology as a predictor of treatment outcome in alcoholics. *Archives of General Psychiatry, 44,* 505–513.

Rouse, S. V., Butcher, J. S., & Miller, K. B. (1999). Assessment of substance abuse in psychotherapy clients: The effectiveness of the MMPI-2 substance abuse scales. *Psychological Assessment, 11,* 101–107.

Salzman, C., Wolfson, A. N., Schatzberg, A., Looper, J., Henke, R., Albanese, M., Schwartz, J., & Miyawaki, E. (1995). Effect of fluoxetine on anger in symptomatic volunteers with borderline personality disorder. *Journal of Clinical Psychopharmacology, 15,* 23–29.

Samenow, S. (1984). *Inside the criminal mind.* New York: Times Books/Random House.

Schooler, N. R. (1995). Integration of family and drug treatment strategies in the treatment of schizophrenia: A selective review. *International Clinical Psychopharmacology, 10,* 73–80.

Schuckit, M. A. (1985). The clinical implications of primary diagnostic groups among alcoholics. *Archives of General Psychiatry, 42,* 1043–1049.

Schuckit, M. A. (1986). Genetic and clinical implications of alcoholism and affective disorder. *American Journal of Psychiatry, 143,* 140–147.

Schuckit, M. A. (1989). Biomedical and genetic markers of alcoholism. In H. W. Goedde & D. P. Agarwal (Eds.), *Alcoholism: Biomedical and genetic aspects.* (pp. 290–302). Elmsford, NY: Pergamon Press.

Schuckit, M. A. (1994). Alcohol and depression: A clinical perspective. *Acta Psychiatrica Scandinavia, 337,* 28–32.

Schuckit, M. A., & Hesselbrock, V. (1994). Alcohol dependence and anxiety disorders: What is the relationship? *American Journal of Psychiatry, 151,* 1723–1735.

Schuckit, M. A., Tipp, J. E., Bergman, B. A., Reich, W., Hesselbrock, V. M., & Smith, T. L. (1997). Comparison of induced and independent major depressive disorders in 2,945 alcoholics. *American Journal of Psychiatry, 154,* 948–957.

Schuckit, M. A., Tipp, J. E., Bucholz, K. K., Nurnberger, J. I. Jr., Hesselbrock, V. M., Crowe, R. R., & Kramer, J. (1997). The life-time rates of three major mood disorders and four major anxiety disorders in alcoholics and controls. *Addiction, 92,* 1289–1304.

Scubiner, H., Tzelepis, A., Isaacson, J. H., Warabasse, L. H., Zacharek, M., & Musial, J. (1995). The dual diagnosis of attention-deficit/hyperactivity disorder and substance abuse: Case reports and literature review. *Journal of Clinical Psychiatry, 56,* 146–150.

Selby, M. J., & Azrin, R. L. (1998). Neuropsychological functioning in drug abusers. *Drug and Alcohol Dependence, 50,* 39–45.

Self, D. W. (1998). Neural substrates of drug craving and relapse in drug addiction. *Annals of Medicine, 30,* 379–389.

Self, D. W., & Nestler, E. J. (1998). Relapse to drug-seeking: Neural and molecular mechanisms. *Drug and Alcohol Dependence, 51,* 49–60.

Sells, S. P. (1998). *Treating the tough adolescent: A family-based, step-by-step guide.* New York: Guilford Press.

Severinghaus, J., & Kinney, J. (1996). Medical management. In J. Kinney (Ed.). *Clinical manual of substance abuse,* (2nd ed. pp. 99–128). St. Louis, MO: Mosby Year Book.

Seyler, M. C. (1971). The Michigan Alcoholism Screening Test: The quest for a new diagnostic instrument. *American Journal of Psychiatry, 127,* 1657–1658.

Shaner, A., Khalsa, M. E., Roberts, L., Wilkins, J., Anglin, D., & Hsieh, S.-C. (1993). Unrecognized cocaine use among schizophrenic patients. *American Journal of Psychiatry, 150,* 758–762.

Shaner, A., Tucker, D. E., Roberts, L. J., & Eckman, T. A. (1999). Disability income, cocaine use and contingency management among patients with cocaine dependence and schizophrenia. In S. T. Higgins & K. Sliverman (Eds.). *Motivating behavior change among illicit-drug abusers: Research on con-*

tingence management interventions (pp. 95–122). Washington, DC: American Psychological Association.

Shearer, S. L. (1994). Dissociative phenomena in women with borderline personality disorder. *American Journal of Psychiatry, 151,* 1324–1328.

Sher, K. J., & Trull, T. J. (1994). Personality and disinhibitory psychopathology: Alcoholism and antisocial personality disorder. *Journal of Abnormal Psychology, 103,* 92–103.

Silk, K. R., Lee, S., Hill, E. M., & Lohr, N. E. (1995). Borderline personality disorder symptoms and severity of sexual abuse. *American Journal of Psychiatry, 152,* 1059–1064.

Slutske, W. S., Heath, A. C., Dinwiddie, S. H., Madden, P. A., Bucholz, K. K., Dunne, M. P., Statham, D. J., & Martin, N. G. (1998). Common genetic risk factors for conduct disorder and alcohol dependence. *Journal of Abnormal Psychology, 107,* 363–374.

Smith, S. S., & Newman, J. P. (1990). Alcohol and drug abuse-dependence disorders in psychopathic and nonpsychopathic criminal offenders. *Journal of Abnormal Psychology, 99,* 430–439.

Sobell, L. C., Toneatto, T., & Sobell, M. B. (1994). Behavioral assessment and treatment planning for alcohol, tobacco and other drug problems: Current status with an emphasis on clinical applications. *Behavior Therapy, 25,* 533–580.

Sokolski, K. N., Cummings, J. L., Abrams, B. I., DeMet, E. M., Katz, L. S., & Costa, J. F. (1994). Effects of substance abuse on hallucination rates and treatment responses in chronic psychiatric patients. *Journal of Clinical Psychiatry, 55,* 380–387.

Solof, P. H. (1994). Is there any drug treatment of choice for the borderline patient? *Acta Psychiatrica Scandinavica Supplement, 379,* 50–55.

Solof, P. H., Lis, J. A., Kelly, T., Cornelius, J., & Ulrich, R. (1994). Risk factors for suicidal behavior in borderline personality disorder. *American Journal of Psychiatry, 151,* 1316–1323.

Sotsky, S. M., Glass, D. R., Shea, M. T., Pilkonis, P. A., Collins, J. F., Elkin, I., Watkins, J. T., Imber, S. D., Leber, W. E., Moyer, J., & Oliveri, M. E. (1991). Patient predictors of response to psychotherapy and pharmacotherapy: Findings in the NIMH Treatment of Depression Collaborative Research Program. *American Journal of Psychiatry, 53,* 283–290.

Spiegel, D. A., & Bruce, T. J. (1997). Benzodiazepines and exposure-based cognitive behavior therapies for panic disorder: Conclusions from combined treatment trials. *American Journal of Psychiatry, 154,* 773–781.

Stark, M. J. (1992). Dropping out of substance abuse treatment: A clinically oriented review. *Clinical Psychology Review, 12,* 93–116.

Stein, D. J., Hollander, E., Decaria, C. M., Simeon, D., Cohen, L., & Aronowitz, B. (1996). m-Chlorophenylpierazine challenge in borderline personality disorder: Relationship of neuroendocrine response, behavioral response and clinical measures. *Biological Psychiatry, 40,* 508–513.

Steinberg, L., Fletcher, A., & Darling, N. (1994). Parental monitoring and peer influences on adolescent substance use. *Pediatrics, 93,* 1060–1064.

Steinglass, P. (1981). The alcoholic family at home: Patterns of interaction in dry, wet and transitional stages of alcoholism. *Archives of General Psychiatry, 38,* 578–584.

Stewart, S. A. (1996). Alcohol abuse in individuals exposed to trauma. *Psychological Bulletin, 120,* 83–112.

Stice, E., Barrera, M., Jr., & Chassin, L. (1998). Prospective differential prediction of adolescent alcohol use and problems use: Examining the mechanisms of effect. *Journal of Abnormal Psychology, 107,* 616–628.

Stone, A. M., Greenstein, R. A., Gamble, G., & McLellan, A. T. (1993). Cocaine use by schizophrenic outpatients who receive depot neuroleptic medication. *Hospital and Community Psychiatry, 44,* 176–177.

Strakowski, S. M., McElroy, S. L., Keck, P. E., Jr., & West, S. A. (1996). The effects of antecedent substance abuse on the development of first-episode psychotic mania. *Journal of Psychiatric Research, 30,* 59–68.

Strub, R. L., & Black, F. W. (1985). *The mental status exam in neurology* (2nd ed.). Philadelphia: Davis.

Svrakic, D. M., & McCallum, K. (1991). Antisocial behavior and personality disorders. *American Journal of Psychotherapy, 45,* 181–197.

Swindle, R. W., Phibbs, C. S., Paradise, M. J., Recine, B. P., & Moos, R. (1995). Inpatient treatment for substance abuse patients with psychiatric disorders: A national study of determinants of readmission. *Journal of Substance Abuse, 7,* 79–97.

Swirsky-Sacchetti, T., Gorton, G., Samuel, S., Sobel, R., Genetta-Wadley, A., & Burleigh, B. (1993). Neuropsychological function in borderline personality disorder. *Journal of Clinical Psychology, 49,* 385–396.

Tarrier, N., Yusupoff, O., Kinney, C., McCarthy, E., Gledhill, A., Haddock, G., & Morris, J. (1998). Randomized controlled trial of intensive cognitive behavior therapy for patients with chronic schizophrenia. *British Medical Journal, 317,* 303–307.

Tarter, R. E., & Vanyukov, M. (1994). Alcoholism: A developmental disorder. *Journal of Consulting and Clinical Psychology, 62,* 1096–1107.

Thase, M. T., Greenhouse, J. B., Frank, E., Reynolds, C. F., III, Pilkonis, P. A., Hurley, K., Grochocinski, V., & Kupfer, D. J. (1997). Treatment of major depression with psychotherapy or psychotherapy-pharmacotherapy combinations. *Archives of General Psychiatry, 54,* 1009–1015.

Thase, M. T., & Kupfer, D. J. (1996). Recent developments in the pharmacotherapy of mood disorders. *Journal of Consulting and Clinical Psychology, 64,* 646–659.

Thase, M. E., Simmons, A. D., & Reynolds, C. F., III. (1996). Significance of abnormal electroencephalographic sleep profiles in major depressions: Association with response to cognitive therapy. *Archives of General Psychiatry, 53,* 99–108.

Thom, B. (1987). Sex differences in help-seeking for alcohol problems: 2. Entry into treatment. *British Journal of Addiction, 82,* 989–997.

Thombs, D. L. (1999). *Introduction to addictive behaviors.* (2nd ed.). New York: Guilford Press.

Tomasson, K., & Vaglum, P. (1996). Psychopathology and alcohol consumption among treatment-seeking alcoholics: A prospective study. *Addiction, 91,* 1019–1030.

Torgersen, S. (1994). Genetics in borderline conditions. *Acta Psychiatrica Scandinavia (Suppl.), 379,* 19–25.

Triffleman, E. G., Marmar, C. R., Delucchi, K. L., & Ronfeldt, H. (1995). Childhood trauma and posttraumatic stress disorder in substance abuse inpatients. *Journal of Nervous and Mental Disease, 183,* 172–176.

Tsuang, D., Cowley, D., Ries, R., Dunner, D., & Roy-Bryne, P. P. (1995). The effects of substance use disorder on the clinical presentation of anxiety and depression in an outpatient psychiatric clinic. *Journal of Clinical Psychiatry, 56,* 549–555.

Tucker, J. A., Vuchinich, R. E., & Gladsjo, J. A. (1994). Environmental events surrounding natural recovery from alcohol-related problems. *Journal of Studies on Alcohol, 55,* 401–411.

Tucker, J. A., Vuchinich, R. E., & Pukish, M. M. (1995). Molar environmental contexts surrounding recovery from alcohol problems by treated and untreated problem drinkers. *Experimental and Clinical Psychopharmacology, 3,* 195–204.

van der Kolk, B. A. (1989). Compulsion to repeat the trauma: Reenactment, revictimization and masochism. *Psychiatric Clinics of North America, 12,* 389–411.

van der Kolk, B. A. (1994). The body keeps score: Memory and the evolving psychobiology of posttraumatic stress. *Harvard Review of Psychiatry, 1,* 253–265.

van Gorp, W. G., Alshuler, L., Theberge, D. C., Wilkins, J., & Dixon, W. (1998). Cognitive impairment in euthymic bipolar patients with and without prior alcohol dependence: A preliminary study. *Archives of General Psychiatry, 55,* 41–46.

van Reekum, R., Links, P. S., Finlayson, M. A., Boyle, M., Boiago, I., Ostrander, L. A., & Moustacalis, E. (1996). Repeat neurobehavioral study of borderline personality disorder. *Journal of Psychiatry and Neurosciences, 21,* 13–20.

Volkow, N. D., Wang, G. J., Iditzeman, R., Fowler, J. S., Overall, J. E., Burr, G., & Wolf, A. P. L. (1994). Recovery of brain glucose metabolism in detoxified alcoholics. *American Journal of Psychiatry, 151,* 178–183.

Waldstein, S. R., Malloy, P. F., Stout, R., & Longabaugh, R. (1996). Predictors of neuropsychological impairment in alcoholics: Antisocial versus nonantisocial subtypes. *Addictive Behavior, 21,* 21–27.

Wallace, J. (1996). Theory of 12-step-oriented treatment. In F. Rotgers, D. S. Keller, & J. Morgenstern (Eds.), *Treating substance abuse: Theory and technique* (pp. 13–36). New York: Guilford Press.

Washton, A. M., & Stone-Washton, N. (1991). *Step zero: Getting to recovery.* Center City, MN: Hazelden.

Wassink, T. H., Flaum, M., Nopoulos, P., & Andreasen, N. C. (1999). Prevalence of depressive symptoms early in the course of schizophrenia. *American Journal of Psychiatry, 156*(2), 315–316.

Watson, C. G., Brown, K. Tilleskjor, C., Jacobs, L., & Purcel, J. (1988). The comparative recidivism rates of voluntary- and coerced-admission male alcoholics. *Journal of Clinical Psychology, 43*, 404–412.

Weaver, T. L., & Clum, G. A. (1993). Early family environments and traumatic experiences associated with borderline personality disorder. *Journal of Consulting and Clinical Psychology, 61*, 1068–1075.

Weisner, C. (1990). The alcohol treatment-seeking process from a problems perspective: Responses to events. *British Journal of Addiction, 85*, 561–569.

Weiss, R. D., Greenfield, S. F., Najavits, L. M., Soto, J. A., Wyner, D., Tohen, M., & Griffin, M. L. (1998). Medication compliance among patients with bipolar disorder and substance use disorder. *Journal of Clinical Psychiatry, 59*, 172–174.

Weiss, R. D., Mirin, S. M., & Griffin, M. L. (1992). Methodological considerations in the diagnosis of coexisting psychiatric disorders in drug abusers. *British Journal of Addiction, 87*, 179–187.

Weiss, R. D., Najavits, L. M., & Greenfield, S. F. (1999). A relapse prevention group for patients with bipolar and substance use disorders. *Journal of Substance Abuse Treatment, 16*, 47–54.

Weiss, R. D., Najavits, L. M., Greenfield, S. F., Soto, J. A., Shaw, S. R., & Wyner, D. (1998). Validity of substance use self-reports in dually diagnosed outpatients. *American Journal of Psychiatry, 155*, 127–128.

Weisz, J. R., Weiss, B., Han, S. S., Granger, D. A., & Morton, T. (1995). Effects of psychotherapy with children and adolescents revisited: A meta-analysis of treatment outcome studies. *Psychological Bulletin, 117*, 450–468.

Wells, E. A., Peterson, P. L., Gainey, R. R., Hawkins, J. D., & Catalano, R. F. (1994). Outpatient treatment for cocaine abuse: A controlled comparison of relapse prevention and 12-step approaches. *American Journal of Drug and Alcohol Abuse, 20*, 1–17.

Wesson, D. R. (Consensus Panel Chair). (1995). *Detoxification from alcohol and other drugs: Treatment improvement protocol (TIP) series.* Rockville, MD: U.S. Department of Health and Human Services. Public Health Service. Substance Abuse and Mental Health Services Administration. Center for Substance Abuse Treatment.

Wilens, T. E., Biederman, J., & Spencer, T. (1996). Attention-deficit hyperactivity disorders and the psychoactive substance use disorders. *Child and Adolescent Psychiatric Clinics of North America, 5*, 73–91.

Wilens, T. E., Biederman, J., Spencer, T. J., & Prince, J. (1995). Pharmacotherapy of adult attention deficit/hyperactivity disorder: A review. *Journal of Clinical Psychopharmacology, 15*, 270–279.

Wills, T. A., McNamara, G., Vaccaro, D., & Hirky, A. E. (1996). Escalated substance use: A longitudinal group analysis from early to middle adolescence. *Journal of Abnormal Psychology, 105*, 166–180.

Wilson, J. P. (1989). *Trauma, transformation and healing: An integrative approach to theory, research and post-traumatic stress therapy.* New York: Brunner/Mazel.

Winokur, G., Coryell, W., Akiskal, H. S., Maser, J. D., Keller, M. B., Endicott, J., & Mueller, T. (1994). Alcoholism in manic–depressive (bipolar) illness:

Familial illness, course of illness and the primary–secondary distinction. *American Journal of Psychiatry, 152*, 365–372.

Wiseman, E. J., Souder, E., & O'Sullivan, P. (1996). Relation of denial of alcohol to neurocognitive impairment and depression. *Psychiatric Services, 47*, 306–308.

Wolf, A. W., Schubert, D. S. P., Patterson, M. B., Grande, T. P., Brocco, K. J., & Pendleton, L. (1998). Associations among psychiatric diagnoses. *Journal of Consulting and Clinical Psychology, 56*, 292–294.

Woodruff, R. A., Guze, S. B., Clayton, P. J. (1972). Anxiety neurosis among psychiatric patients. *Comprehensive Psychiatry, 13*, 165–170.

Woody, G. E., McLellan, A. T., & Luborsky, L. (1984). Psychiatric severity as a predictor of benefits from psychotherapy. *American Journal of Psychiatry, 141*, 1171–1177.

Woody, G. E., O'Brien, C. P., McLellan, A. T., & Evans, B. D. (1982). Use of antidepressants along with methadone in maintenance patients. *Annals of the New York Academy of Sciences, 398*, 120–127.

Yoshioka, M. R., Thomas, E. J., & Ager, R. D. (1992). Nagging and other drinking control efforts of spouses of uncooperative alcohol abusers: Assessment and modification. *Journal of Substance Abuse, 4*, 309–318.

Index